HOW CAN I
TALK IF MY
LIPS DON'T
MOVE?

Also by Tito Rajarshi Mukhopadhyay

The Mind Tree
The Gold of the Sunbeams

HOW CAN I TALK IF MY LIPS DON'T MOVE?

inside my autistic mind

TITO RAJARSHI MUKHOPADHYAY

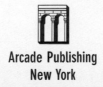

Arcade Publishing
New York

FIRST EDITION

Library of Congress Cataloging-in-Publication Data
Mukhopadhyay, Tito Rajarshi.
  How can I talk if my lips don't move? : inside my autistic mind / Tito Rajarshi Mukhopadhyay. —1st ed.
     p. cm.
  ISBN 978-1-55970-859-3 (alk. paper)
  I. Mukhopadhyay, Tito Rajarshi—Mental health. 2. Autistic youth—United States—Biography. I. Title.

  RJ506.A9M85 2008
  618.92'85882—dc22   2007022842

Published in the United States by Arcade Publishing, Inc., New York
Distributed by Hachette Book Group USA

Visit our Web site at www.arcadepub.com

10 9 8 7 6 5 4 3 2 I

Designed by API

EB

PRINTED IN THE UNITED STATES OF AMERICA

To you who think my words matter

Contents

Foreword

What do we really know about how children, adolescents, and adults with autism obtain and process information? What do we, the "neurotypicals," know about how autistic individuals see and interpret their world? In 1986 Temple Grandin published her first book, *Emergence*, in which she described growing up with autism, providing for the first time an insider's view of a different kind of life. Since then, a growing number of similar personal accounts have appeared, each adding more insight into the inner world of autistics. This book is yet another personal story, but what makes this one so remarkable is that it comes from a young man whose verbal expressive language is profoundly impaired but who communicates almost exclusively by independently writing or typing his thoughts and ideas on a computer.

Autism is a behaviorally defined disorder characterized by impaired social interaction, delayed and disordered language, and isolated areas of interest. First described in 1943 by Dr. Leo Kanner, autism is believed to be largely genetic in etiology, but environmental factors are also suspected of playing a role. Current prevalence rates suggest that 1 in every 150 children is affected, with a male-to-female ratio of 4 to 1. It is now recognized that autism is clinically heterogeneous, and although a core cluster of features unites those affected, there can be wide variations in presentation, associated symptoms, and severity. This variability and the likelihood that autism may have multiple etiologies have resulted in the term autism spectrum disorders (ASD), which is now in common usage.

Basic scientific research in autism is moving forward ever more rapidly, parallel to and in association with active clinical research, but much remains to be learned. Attending to the observations of those affected with the disorder can help us frame realistic and meaningful questions worthy of investigation. For example, Tito tells us about his reliance on sensory associations to help him process information more efficiently. Although there is a good deal of interest in sensory modulation dysfunction in autism, relatively little research addresses sensory processing in this disorder. Tito also tells us that he needs multiple repeat visits or exposures to specific environments to become comfortable, and that once comfortable, he comes to enjoy the experience and eventually becomes "addicted" to it. What might that observation tell us about the underlying neurobiology of developing familiarity and the ability or inability to deal with novelty? There has been significant interest and research in face processing. Tito tells us that when he was younger, he could not look at faces because he felt threatened by them. He found faces difficult to decipher, which frequently led to mix-ups in identification, causing him to appear impolite. However, if he heard the voice of the person in question and could match that voice to the face and to a past event, he could then identify the person. Thus, Tito tells us that he relies on multiple modalities to accurately identify people he has met previously, suggesting a possible dysfunction with data gathering and cross-modal memory.

Each one of Tito's observations in this book affords us an opportunity to consider how this young man is taking in and handling information in a variety of modalities. He tells us that throughout his life, his mother utilized every circumstance, opportunity, and event to teach through experience, explanation, drawing, and writing. There is little doubt that Tito is who he is in large part because of the persistence and dedication of his mother and her ever-present and creative teaching. At the end of the book, Tito considers his future. He wonders whether he will be able to live independently someday and ponders on what his contribution to the world may be when he is older. Whatever the future holds for Tito, he has already made a significant contribution to the field of autism. Here we have a young man who is essentially non-verbal but who clearly is very intelligent and poetic. While he may perceive the world differently, his observations and experiences are critically important, and we can learn much from him. We now know that an autistic person who is unable to speak does not necessarily have nothing to say. Tito forces us to think beyond the obvious, and that in and of itself is an important lesson. Thank you, Tito, for writing this book and for sharing some of your thoughts with those of us who are clinicians, scientists, parents, professionals, and therapists. May your future be bright, and may you continue to help us all to ask questions and to find the answers to autism.

Margaret L. Bauman, M.D., Ph.D.
Director, Autism Research Foundation

Author's Note

There are times in everyone's life when there is a need to tell a story. It can be any story. It can be a story about a hairpin you were fascinated by, on someone's hair, whose name you will never know, but who had inspired you to wait at the same bus stop for seven straight evenings in the hope of seeing just one glimpse of her, and in the end giving up. Then you end up writing a page of poems dedicated to her.

A story can be about the shadow of a beggar woman on some street in Bangalore, when I saw her scratch her head of tangled white hair under a hot midday sun, in the hope of getting some coins from passersby. A story of a hope to survive.

A story can be about the mask of a tribal dancer, who is proud of being the last representative of his dying race because of cultural diffusion and global tendencies toward modernization, as he claimed.

Or a story could grow around a hat, which you saw on a large head and knew at once that the hat and head were made for each other.

This is how I grew my stories, from this and that, now and then, here or there, to compose this book.

**HOW CAN I
TALK IF MY
LIPS DON'T
MOVE?**

Through the Mirror

Right now, I am thinking about a mirror. It was a mirror in one of the rooms upstairs, in the house where I spent my second and third years of life. The mirror was in front of a window, and it reflected the rocks of those sun-baked hills outside the window. I would stand in front of that mirror, not to admire the landscape in its reflection. I would not stand in front of it to see how well my hair was groomed either. I would stand in front of it because I believed that the mirror wanted to tell me a story. And I believed that the mirror wanted to tell me a story because I wanted to tell *it* a story. I would tell my story to the mirror, and the mirror would tell me back the story. I would think about a tilted sky surrounding those climbing goats on the hill. I would believe that the mirror heard my thoughts and would show me the tilted sky.

I was not able to talk when I was two or three years old. My stories were not meant for human ears. Human ears cannot hear anything other than sounds. But not my ears, as I believed then. And not the ears of the mirror either. I believed that if you cared enough to listen, you could hear the sky and earth speaking to each other in the language of blue and brown. And I believed that if you cared enough to listen, you could hear the walls of the room you were in, telling the floor not to stare at them, while the floor wondered, "Where else should I look?"

A language of white and red. The white of the walls and the red of the painted cement floor. The mirror heard everything. I knew that the mirror heard everything because only when I stood in front of it could I hear the walls and floor talk. Otherwise, why should I stand in front of it and wait for the open window to sing to the walls in the color of air? Only after I heard the silent voices, could I tell my story to the mirror. Stories with sounds of blue, white, red, or brown. Or stories with the colors of air.

One day, while I stood in front of it, I realized that it was easy to go through it and come out through it. And I realized that I could go in or come out only when the world behind me became transparent. Absolutely transparent. And where would all the colors of the world behind me go? I realized that the mirror would absorb all the colors within its own stretch of self. The blue sky behind the window would look bluer in the mirror. The sun-baked hills would turn browner in it. And I would look behind me to see the real sky and hill. I would be surprised to see them, colored with the color of air.

Stories waited for me behind the mirror. So I was needed on its other side. There was no great trouble to go through the mirror to the other side. All I needed to do was to stare intensely at any shadow on the corner of the wall as it was reflected in my eyes.

Voices of colors
And voices of shadows
Voices of movement
And their echoes
Voices of silence
Spun near or far
Through spaces and distance
Soaking my ears.

The Color of Basic Words

Real voices. I could be waiting behind a shadow listening to a story in red and green, when I would be interrupted by a real voice made of sound, thus dissolving the story of red and green. And then, to my utter horror, I would find myself surrounded by real voices. Voices made of sounds, on the real side of the mirror. The mirror would never reflect voices made of sounds. I, however, knew that it could if it tried hard enough.

"If you try hard enough, you can talk," Mother's voice would tell me. Mother's voice would tell me that when no one was around and when she took a break from singing the same song many times over because if she didn't, I would threaten a temper tantrum. Mother had to be careful that no one was around because she did not want those women to smile at her for trying to explain things to a boy who had not even learned how to talk yet. Their smiles were the color of jaundice yellow, and that yellow was so dense, every color could be choked by its strength. I believed that Mother saw what I saw. And I believed that she was careful because she did not want to be choked by jaundice yellow either.

"You need to talk basic words to him first," those voices

would tell Mother. Basic words included a series of *dada*, *mama*, *kaka*, *baba*, and so on.

"Only after he masters those words, will he be able to follow explanations like, 'Try hard to talk.'" I would hear their words in their voices of jaundice yellow.

I wondered which colors would go with basic words like *dada*, *mama*, *kaka*, and *baba*. So I would stand in front of the mirror and mentally say those basic words and wait for the mirror to show me their colors reflected in it. I soon realized that the mirror could not reflect the colors of those basic words.

"Only after it masters how to reflect the basic words, will it be able to follow other explanations like, 'Try hard to reflect,'" I concluded.

The Color of My Scream

Many times, in the midst of other sounds, I could hear my own voice, laughing or screaming. The mirror never could color those sounds. Whenever I heard real sounds, I stopped to see the stories forming behind the mirror. My hearing became increasingly powerful whenever that happened, and I stopped seeing anything. I could focus all my concentration on only one sense, and that is hearing. I am not sure whether or not I had to put any kind of effort toward hearing because I was too young and uninformed in science to analyze the sensory battle that was taking place within my nervous system. It just meant that my colors would disappear if there were sounds vibrating around me.

Was I scared or confused? I am not certain, as I did not know what the rules of the world were and what other people experienced. I concluded that everybody and everything, including the maid who had to move me away from the mirror, experienced what I did.

The maid had to move me away from the mirror because I did not move when she asked me, "Tito baba, please move a little, as I have to mop the floor." The sound of her voice made me come back from behind the mirror while I was hearing a story of green and red from the green of the curtains and the red of the cement floor, which the maid intended to mop. The smell of phenol water from her bucket and mop filled the spaces which were yet to be filled with stories of green and red.

One experience diffused into the next. And every experience settled in my mind as an example of a natural phenomenon, which laid down the rules of the world. For instance, if I saw a bird on a tree, and, at that very moment, I saw someone walking across the street in front of our gate, I concluded that every time a bird sits on a tree, someone needs to walk across the street.

What if they did not happen together? Well, I would panic and get so anxious that I would scream. Screaming would stop me from looking at the tree or looking at the street, for I can do only one thing at a time. I can either use my eyes or use my ears. Hearing my voice screaming would stop my eyes from looking.

"Why is he screaming?" voices would ask Mother. "She should know. After all, she is his mother."

Mother would give them some reason. She would say that I was hungry, or she would say that I was hot. She would say that I must have been bitten by fire ants because they were all over the yard, or she would say that I was tired. Then she would rush me inside to find out for herself why I was screaming.

"There, there, let me rub your feet with cold water. Those bad, bad fire ants!" Mother's voice would continue to distract me while I heard my voice scream. I would scream, and I would wonder. I would wonder about the mirror upstairs. I was sure that it was forming a story in red and green once again. The red of fire ants and the green of grass. My voice would scream, and I would wonder whether the mirror upstairs was aware of my screaming. I would lose all control over my screaming voice, and would wonder when it would stop. My voice would scream, and I would realize Mother's voice was singing something familiar in my ear. I would slowly concentrate on the words of her song and try to mentally sing along because she repeated most of her songs so often to me that I had them memorized. After listening to the words of her song, I would wonder why I could no longer hear my voice screaming. And, to my relief, I would realize that my voice had stopped screaming. I would continue to think about the mirror. Surely it could reflect the sound of a scream. Mother's voice would begin to fade out the more I thought about the mirror, and the urge to stand in front of it would fill my whole concentration. I would hurry and rush upstairs, like a dedicated student who had heard the school bell ring.

I would rush upstairs only to realize that Mother was following me with her voice, continuing her song. Mother's voice fading out, like some distant memory, going farther away, yet not leaving me completely. There was no way I could tell her to stop following me because I did not have a talking voice then. There was no way I could tell her that the mirror would not show me any red or green story if there was so much distraction from her voice.

Following the Belief

Mother had a strange belief then. If she talked continuously to me, I would begin to talk. So she followed me around with her voice and with her belief, like a faithful believer following some faith.

If people were present, they would hear her counting the steps on the staircase as we climbed. They would hear her tell me to be careful and not go so fast. They would hear her tell me that the staircase was red because the floor was made of red cement. And they would hear her tell me that the stairs were rectangular in shape.

Mother followed me around with her voice, explaining every detail of my actions and defining my surroundings. Mother made it a point to tell me that I was climbing because I was moving away from the ground. She never failed to explain that it was my legs that helped me climb, if I cared to know. Every aspect of climbing was explained by her voice in great detail every time I would go upstairs in the hope of some quiet time with the mirror.

Was she even concerned about whether or not I listened or understood her? Probably not. She was extremely talkative when she knew that no one was watching to comment on her efforts with me.

I memorized her words because of the repetition. Before I was even five years old, I could define the words *gravity*, *force*, and *acceleration* because Mother defined them to me with dedicated constancy.

I would finally reach the mirror in the hope of seeing a story and in the hope of some silence. But with Mother standing behind me, I could only hear her voice telling me that I had two eyes, and these were my eyes, and when I close them I cannot see. "And just have a good look at our noses! Aren't they alike?"

Mother told me the story of Snow White and her stepmother, the queen, who would ask her mirror every day the status of her beauty. Mother told me the story many times, making me wonder what color the word *beauty* would be. I had associated it with women in general, without actually knowing the essence of it. I thought women possessed some kind of object called "beauty," and Snow White's stepmother, the queen, had a bigger object called "beauty," compared to other women. And I had the belief that mirrors that talked knew who had the biggest object called "beauty."

The mirror upstairs was silent. I waited for it to say the basic words first, like *baba*, *kaka*, *mama*, and *dada*. And people around me waited for me to begin speaking my basic words.

Mother gave me a little handheld mirror through which I could see anything I wanted to. She took it with her whenever she followed me out to the garden with her voice. She followed me in and out with her voice and the handheld mirror. She tried to see what I was looking at and reflect that in the mirror. I would look up and hear her voice narrating to me what I was probably looking at. I could hear her voice telling me that it was the sky I was looking at and it is blue. And if I was really interested in what type of blue the sky was, she would be more than willing to tell me that it was azure, a special type of blue. Her voice continued to explain that in Bengali sky is *Aakash*. Fancy that! So as I was looking at who knows what, I was memorizing her words, which revolved around the sky. And because her voice would not leave me alone, explaining to me, her three-year-old son, the presence of oxygen and nitrogen in the air, I memorized that, too. For it was not once or twice that she uttered her sky lesson, following me with her voice and the handheld mirror, but several times a day and many times a week. So I knew what the planets were and what the Milky Way was.

Did I realize that I was learning? I do not think so because after a while, I expected her to narrate her lessons and sort of knew what she would tell me, for it had become a habit. She would tell me, "Now let's look at the sky through this handheld mirror. But if we turn our heads too fast, how are we going to see the sky? Never mind, now let's see what is so interesting in that corner where you're looking. Corners can be very interesting, especially when they are between two straight lines. . . ." I knew she would tell me about angles.

Mother knew nothing about my selective vision when I was three. I could look at certain things but not at others. Things that calmed my senses were easier to see, while things that stressed my vision were not easy to look at. So perhaps I could not see things as people expected me to see.

I could not feel comfortable, seeing the sky or corners or anything through the little handheld mirror. I would walk back to the house, giving back the little handheld mirror to her because I did not want it. I had no way to make her understand that the mirror upstairs was different from the little handheld mirror. She would not understand even if I tried to look away from the mirror.

"If you love looking at the big mirror, why don't you love looking at this mirror?" Mother's voice wanted to know. "And if you compare real objects and their reflected images upstairs, you should compare them with this mirror, too." Mother was determined to make me accept the little mirror. So she would bring the little handheld mirror as close as possible to my face, so that my real nose would touch the reflected nose. Then she would make a "nose touching" game with the small mirror.

"Here comes your nose again," as she slowly brought the handheld mirror close to my face. Then she would move it away all of a sudden with, "Here it goes back again."

I think I was supposed to laugh at the mirror play or whatever she wanted me to think it was. Later, when I observed children, not through the eyes of the mirror but through my own reason and understanding, I realized that when there is something intense going on, there is an expectation of some kind of response. So perhaps Mother expected me to laugh at the mirror that was coming near me, touching my nose, and moving away from my nose, along with her animated voice. I never responded. I was not interested in the nose reflection game.

More than the reflections, I was interested in the essence of the reflected objects and the possible stories about them. I never liked to be away from the upstairs mirror for long. As if my thoughts would only flow if I was near it. Some days I thought of nothing else than the mirror upstairs.

What Could the Upstairs Mirror
Tell the Handheld Mirror?

With her handheld mirror, Mother showed me tricks with mirrors facing each other, forming an infinite number of reflections. Something I love to see at a barber's shop now. I could see an infinite number of reflected windows, and all that I could see through the window was reflected an infinite number of times when two mirrors faced each other in parallel positions. I saw the two mirrors interact with each other, not in any language of blue, white, yellow, or brown but in a completely new language. They interacted in the language of reflections, something that they would not share with me. I could not understand their language, but I could appreciate it. I was fascinated by this new language of reflection and intimacy between the two mirrors. I wondered about all the secret stories they shared between them, like relatives talking about their family, reflection replying to reflection. I wondered about those stories and their who-knows-what secrets, which I was not a part of.

Did I want to learn their language? I do not think so. For there are many things in this world that are beautiful, but much of them remains a secret to us. A woman looks beautiful because she is covered by her skin. If I was exposed to her anatomy with her muscles, bones, and vital organs, I might cease to see her beauty.

I took the handheld mirror from Mother. For many days, I would face one mirror to another and guess what they were telling each other. Perhaps they were comparing each other's reflections, as blue was reflected by blue and was further reflected by more blue. I wondered about their secret interactions. I built my own stories about their communications. Sometimes I made those colors dispute each other. Sometimes I made the colors share their secrets with the wind.

No Wonder I Don't Talk!

One day I happened to realize that when people moved their lips, they made a talking sound known as voice. I happened to see Mother's lips move when she sang to me. For the next few days I would go upstairs, and stand in front of the mirror in the hope of seeing my lips move. I had every bit of patience with the mirror, and the mirror had every bit of patience with me.

I could see the green curtains move with the breeze from the windows. I could see the leaves of the sal-trees move, and I could see the ceiling fan move. They moved in front and behind the mirror. Even my hands moved when I flapped them. Only my lips would not move.

"No wonder I don't talk. How am I going to talk if my lips don't move? Strange! People don't understand such a simple fact!" I was talking to the mirror and heard my words echo back with the air of the ceiling fan to let me know that the mirror understood exactly what I was trying to explain.

"And why wouldn't the mirror talk? It would not talk, simply because it had no lips to move." I had to explain it in case it wondered, too.

Many a day after that I could hear people who could

move their lips and who had voices ask Mother why I had not begun to talk. "What, he is almost three and still does not talk?"

Someone gave Mother a recipe that made her nephew talk. "Give him honey mixed with ginger every morning."

Someone else had a different opinion. "Give him lemon peels mixed with margossa leaf paste." That was exactly what someone gave someone's neighbor's grandson who would not talk even after he turned four. "Today that grandson is a father of two!"

"Nature is a remedy in itself." Someone else suggested how fresh air could be a great help for the lungs, which needed to puff out air in order to produce the voice.

I would stand before the mirror. I would stand before the mirror with echoes of those remedies and with my still lips. I would stand before the mirror with a thoughtful mind, thinking about a moment when I would consume enough honey and ginger or lemon peel and margossa leaf paste or breathe in fresh air from Nature's own remedy and see my lips move.

My thoughtful mind would wonder about the sound of my talking voice, which I could only hear when I laughed or screamed. I promised the mirror that I would remember not to distract it with all my talking, especially when it showed me stories of wind and the ceiling fan in the color of air, or when it showed me the story of the curtains and the window in the colors of sunlight and green. I promised the mirror with complete sincerity. The mirror reflected back my promise with total earnestness.

> And all my mirror tales are gone
> As my life goes on and on
> Through my age, yet stories follow
> Into the world of my shadow.

Shadows Don't Tell Stories

My shadow, I believed, was my greatest companion. Every time I stood under the sun, out in the yard, along with the shadows of those tall sal-trees, every time I walked inside the house and Mother switched on the lights, even though it was daytime, because I would scream if she did not, and every time I walked in the streets under the light of the streetlamps during summer evenings, I found my shadow.

I would see my shadow in various sizes, sometimes long and sometimes short. I would wonder what it meant when it grew long and what it meant when it grew short. I knew that it would not tell me anything. It would not tell me the reason because I would not ask it. And I would not ask it because I could not talk. And how could I talk when my lips would not move?

However, I found out that even if I could not control its size, I could at least control its actions. For it was bound to do exactly what I did. It would jump or run only if I wanted it to. Sometimes I had this feeling that it wanted to walk, but I did not let it do so because I wanted to teach it some discipline. "You can't get all that you want all the time," I meant to tell it when I thought it was getting too impatient for a walk.

Another day I continued to jump up and down on the verandah, only to give my shadow some exercise. I would not stop jumping up and down, even though Mother was trying to distract me, not realizing that my shadow needed some exercise.

The streetlamp in front of the house helped form the shadow on the verandah wall at the entrance of our house. The streetlamp formed other shadows, too. And Mother's shadow hand was putting deep pressure on my shadow shoulder. I saw my shadow stop jumping. Then I realized that my shadow stopped jumping because I had stopped jumping.

Shadows never told any story.
Many times I waited for my shadow to begin some story.
But my shadow never told me any story.
I wondered why.
And I wondered why not.
I wondered why
Shadows don't tell stories.

I came up with an answer after much thought. "How would a shadow tell a story without having a color of its own?"

All the time shadows had to borrow the colors of the objects on which they would fall. And they colored all objects in one universal color. That color is the color of a shadow, which is a darker color on the borrowed color. I could now imagine how a shadow could silence the interaction between other colors if those colors happened to fall in the territory of its silence.

I could see the night jasmines wet with morning dew, lit with fresh sunshine, trying to form a story in white with their jasmine-petal smell. I would see the story spread in the air. Then I would put my hands above it, so that my hands cast a shadow on the flowers. I would see that the moment I put my shadow above the flowers, the story would immediately stop forming. I would imagine the white of the petals and the wet jasmine smell waiting to be freed from the bond of the shadow of my hands, so I would move my hands away from them. Immediately I could imagine the story beginning to form. Perhaps I would touch other flowers like those yellow ixoras with my shadow.

My boundary between imagining and experiencing something was a very delicate one. Perhaps it still is. So many times I need to cross-check with Mother, or someone who can understand my voice now, whether an incident really happened around my body or presence.

Flapping My Hands,
Flapping My Shadow

My hands had made a connection with my shadow. They would begin to flap excitedly at the sight of my shadow, while my eyes would fixate on the effect of their melting shapes, as they moved faster and faster, along with their shadows on the wall, on the floor, or anywhere. I would charm my eyes as I would see my hands becoming transparent as they moved faster and faster, ready to become so transparent as if to challenge their shadows, "How would you shape me now?"

Stories passed in and out of the transparency of my flapping hands. Although the mirror could not be around those stories all the time, and although I could not form or find any story with my hands moving so fast to continue forming the transparency, I knew that all the stories had collected around my flapping hands ready to play an in-and-out game with my fingers.

Stories of the wall, stories covered with smells coming from the kitchen, and stories of nothing covered with the colors of the shadow began to play in-and-out games with the fingers of my flapping hands. To make them pass through my fingers, I needed to continue flapping and maintain their transparency with my speed. I looked at the transparency created by my flapping hands. I wondered how many stories would pass in and out of that transparency. Although I was not able to count in a regular manner then because I was not taught how to, I still kept count. I kept count in threes.

I kept count in threes because when anyone like Mother or my father asked me to jump or begin some action like running or going up the stairs, or climbing on their backs and they would act as my horse, and I would be a gallant rider, they would begin by saying, "Here we go . . . one . . . two and-and-and . . . three!" in a very ritualistic manner, making me anticipate the final number "three."

I was so entertained and impressed by the finality of "three" that I would count everything in threes. My belief in the three count was further strengthened when I looked up at the ceiling fans in all the rooms. The ceiling fans in our house had three blades. Every time I entered a room, I would look up at their blades and count, "One . . . two . . . and . . . and . . . three," just as Mother's voice and Father's voice said in my mind.

Of course I heard the rest of the numbers that followed three from Mother's voice, because she would count the stairs as she followed me upstairs whenever she realized that I was heading for the mirror. Never in those early years did I asso-ciate the numbers following three to my counting the stories, which I believed went in and out of my fingers or my flapping hands.

Autism! A Fancy Word

"Does he flap his hands all the time?" the clinical psychologist in a Calcutta hospital asked Mother.

There were wooden cupboards all around the room, stuck to the walls, which had glass doors. And those glass doors reflected everything. Although they were not as good as the mirror, I thought they would do for the time being, while Mother's voice and the clinical psychologist's voice discussed my hands. Those glass doors reflected the chairs, tables, wide windows, the lamps, the old high ceiling fans, shadows, and people as shadowed shapes. They also reflected my flapping hands. I was impressed. "Every room in this world needs glass doors!"

I chose to stand in the corner between two glass doors, so that I could see as many reflections of my flapping hands as possible through the glass. There were toys and wooden blocks in those cupboards. I was not interested in them. I was not interested in things I did not know how to use. I remember the doors of the cupboards opening, while I tried to move myself along with the door because I wanted to continue seeing the reflections of that wonder room through the glass doors.

I was invited several times to approach all those blocks and toys that were now laid on the table and do something with them. I could either pile them up, or I could line them up. I could shake them, or I could push them and play a train game. I could do anything I wanted with them, so that the clinical psychologist could record it in her observation chart.

I remember the encouraging voices of Mother and the clinical psychologist tempting me, asking me, prodding me, and coaxing me to come to the table and start playing. Mother brought me to the table once or twice, so that I could do something with those toys. And each time I was brought near the table, I would go back to stand in front of the cupboards. How could I tell them that the shadows and reflections made me feel secure? I knew exactly what to expect from them. I did not know what to expect from those toys.

I remember the clinical psychologist writing down or, rather, hearing her write down something in her chart (which later I was told by Mother when she and I could converse was the word *non-response*). And because I flapped my hands, because I did not respond to those blocks, because I did not talk, and because I could not imitate her, the diagnosis: autism.

Autism! A fancy word. Well, now that I knew I was autistic, I began to group things under it. I made up a whole list of things that I thought had autism. The curtains that moved in the wind, the big and small leaves that moved a little more with the air because of their suspended positions, the little bits of paper, or the pages of an open book under a fan were classified as autistic. They were affected with autism because they flapped, because they would not respond to any blocks, because they did not talk, and I was sure that they would not be able to imitate the clinical psychologist. I wondered how the clinical psychologist would look if she imitated the leaves on a branch if the leaves wanted to find out about her condition.

I finally knew the reason why I would not talk. It was because I was autistic. I wished to tell the curtains and the leaves that they, too, were autistic.

My shadow followed me around, blocking stories as it always did with its greater story of nothingness.

"Once there was an autistic red," I thought the mirror upstairs was showing me. I was about to see more when my shadow stole every view of that story, and red became a shadow red, with no story. It was no longer a fancy autistic red.

Shadows the Color of My Scream!

I would sometimes wake up in the middle of the night and look around for my shadow. I did not realize then, when I was two or three years old, that night brings with it its own greater shadow, which can cover all the other shadows within its enormous stretch of sleep.

I remember my voice screaming when I could not see my shadow anywhere around me. I wondered whether it had left me here all alone. I was afraid that I would lose my existence because my shadow had left me. I thought and believed that my shadow was an extension of my body. The feeling of losing my shadow was like losing a part of my body.

I remember Mother trying to hold me and walk up and down the semi-lit rooms, softly singing in my ear. She was scared that I would wake the neighbors. My scream would stretch in the darkness slowly, beginning to color its blackness with the color of my scream. And then it became my business to color every part of the night with the color of my scream.

> There was Mother's voice,
> Trickling down with drops of a tune.
> There was the floating depth

Of some thought-filled dark.
There were sleeping eyes
Lit with voices of dreams.
As I saw them all
With the color of my scream.
Mother's voice trickled the tune
Drop by drop.
As I heard her voice in my ears
Subdued and soft.
Every drop with a color
In every word,
I saw the color of my scream fade
Perhaps I had stopped.

Tracing the Shape of Shadows and Trapping Them in Place

When I grew older and learned to hold a pencil, Mother taught me how to trace the outlines of shadows. She gave me a chalk stick and taught me how to trace the outlines of the shadows of my arms, legs, and hands on the cement floor. As I did so, I started seeing shadows in a new light. I could now trap their shapes within the boundaries of my chalk tracing. Those traced shapes remained there on the floor long after I had moved my hands away from those spots, like pieces of my own history. And as I watched the maid mopping them out with phenol water, I could see them getting wiped away by one sweep of her mop. But I was not hurt to see those shapes go. For I had the power of the remaining chalk piece in my hands, and the floor stretched clean in front of me, waiting for my next mark.

I traced shadows of anything I saw as part of my duty, once I got good at tracing.

And Mother encouraged me by projecting vegetable shadows on the floor. For example, she would hold potatoes and onions or cauliflowers and cabbages up against the sunlight during the day, or bulb light during the evenings, so that I could trace all of their shadows on the verandah cement with my chalk stick.

Sometimes in the evenings, when sunlight had long faded out and streetlamps were lit up in front of our house, their glow from the open windows fell on the red cement floor in the drawing room because Mother would turn off the light in the room, so that the monsoon bugs would stay out of the house. Monsoon bugs were always drawn toward the light. They would stay who knows where during the day. But after dusk they would come out in swarms and invade the houses if they saw light. And what would they do? Nothing but fly around and around the light in the room. And they would fly and knock against faces, or sit on your cheek or arm, waiting for you to squish them. No one needed them at home. But once they were drawn toward the streetlamps, you could be sure that they would stay there. And once they stayed there, you could go ahead and turn on the lights.

The glow from the streetlamps would come in through the windows, so that the shape of the window would fall on the floor. I would trace the outline of the window as it fell on the floor. Mother would mop it, and I would redraw it.

I would seek out new stories in those shapes on the floor. Sometimes there were too many shapes on the floor, crowded by each other's outlines, making one wonder which line or which curve belonged to which shadow, making it look like a whole floor area of confusion.

I wondered about the whole chalk-mark area of confused scribbles. "What would they think about themselves if they happened to look at themselves in the mirror? Would they recognize their own shapes and know whose shadows they were?" And as I wondered, I could hear myself laugh or breathe very loud. Perhaps I would hear Mother in the kitchen with the sound of pots or the water tap turned on. Whatever I heard at that instant, I imagined it as the voice of confusion. "It must be the confused voice of those crowded chalk marks on the floor."

Although shadows did not have any story to tell, I consoled my mind that at least their chalk-mark tracings did. Some had the voices of my laughter, others had the voices of the water tap, while some had the voices of those heavy stainless-steel pots.

I leave my shadow story behind
In some yonder way back time
As they shade here and there
On my front or anywhere.
Shadows of day under shade of sun

TITO RAJARSHI MUKHOPADHYAY

Day by day they all return.
Shadows of night lit by stars
Fill my sleep or waking hours.

My Story Forms around Staircases

Staircases filled me with wonder because I saw my shadow splitting up into different vertical and horizontal planes as I climbed up and down them. I would wish for a staircase that would let me climb through my waking hours. I wished that it could lead me to some place, which would be filled with shadows and mirrors or whatever wonders it could offer. I was ready for any wonder. It did not matter what it was. For only through those wonder experiences would I be able to build my memory.

I would remember a wall not by its flatness but because of a nail that had cast its shadow under the overhead light. And because of that nail, I would imagine and grow my probable stories around it. Stories of a clock or a picture hanging from that nail covering up the place where the shadow was cast. Or stories of a wall chandelier or perhaps a birthday balloon tied to that nail. And anything that would hang from that nail would mark the character on the wall and give my mind its wonder experience so that through it I would store the memory of that wall. Otherwise, a wall would be just any wall, like anybody being anybody.

Since there was no such wonder staircase, and since there

was no such place filled with shadows and mirrors, I began to mentally climb the imagined staircase. I climbed and I climbed to who knows where. I climbed with my shadow in front of me, broken by alternate vertical and horizontal planes, leading me somewhere.

> Thus I climbed up through passages of heaven
> Or I climbed up through tunnels of hell
> Or I climbed through here or there
> I am not sure for yet I cannot tell
> Shadows on those stairs followed my feet
> I heard nothing else but footsteps and heartbeats.

Whenever or wherever I saw staircases, I thought they were meant for me to climb.

Railway Staircases

Railway stations in India have overpasses between two platforms, under which trains could go to and fro. I was fascinated by those overpasses. While waiting for our train, I would climb up and down, up and down, the staircases of the overpasses. Mother would try to show me the trains and other interesting happenings that took place around us on the platforms.

"Did you see that old compartment waiting like a lonely old man?" She would try to turn my head in some direction. Or "Did you see how that porter is trying to lift that heavy suitcase while balancing a bed-holder on his head?" She would point in another direction, perhaps in the direction of the porter.

> I saw it perhaps, or I saw it not
> I saw nothing but the staircases
> Yet I gathered all that went around
> From what she described and what she said.

With my busy feet, I climbed up and down the staircases of those overpasses, while Mother's voice continued to describe how the porter, in his red uniform, dropped a fruit basket because he was in such a hurry and how the owner of that basket was scolding the poor, embarrassed, half-fed porter who was being humiliated despite his apologies.

Train passengers in India need to carry many things for a railway journey. So they need porters. And porters need passengers, because they need work. Most passengers carry their bedding, their food, and their big water carriers, which would last at least a day if they are economical with it. Then they carry fruit and snack baskets because who knows what food will be available in those states of India through which their trains will pass. For people of one state usually prefer to stick to the food of their own state as long as possible, even while they travel. So people brought lunch-carriers, packed with home-cooked food for their journey. Families, babies, luggage, and food stuck close together under the roof of the Indian railway platform, with patience and pride.

I climbed up or down, wondering what the shadow of that fruit basket would be like and what the mirror back home had to say about it. And as I wondered, Mother would begin her next description about those flies following a candy vendor. I could hear Mother's voice, the hawking vendors, the whistle of an engine, and the whole voice of the platform, alive with flies, dust, confusion, and people. And while I wondered what those flies would think about climbing the staircases with me, I also wondered about their little shadows. "Could their shadows keep up with their speed?"

I climbed up and down with my dutiful air, as if that was what I was supposed to do. And Mother would continue on with her narration of the events around us with her dutiful air, as if that was what she was supposed to do.

Sometimes she told me she saw a large turban on someone's small head. She told me that the turban was parrot green in color. And she told me that it was the brightest of all the colors she could see on the platform. Mother continued her narration with her own opinion about the owner of the large parrot green turban and small head. "He sure had a great appreciation for color," she observed. "Otherwise, why would he wear an oxblood red shirt with the parrot green turban?"

I wondered about a red and green story, and wished that the mirror back home got to see it. A story about parrot green and oxblood red. But before I could think of one, Mother announced that a beggar was heading toward us.

I climbed up and down those overpass staircases, wishing that it could be our home. And while I would wish, while I would hear Mother, and while I would climb, our train would come and Mother would drag me away from those staircases toward the train because my reluctant feet would not want to leave those staircases.

Why Was Mother Stopping Me from Climbing?

I once had a temper tantrum. I had a temper tantrum in a doctor's clinic. The doctor's clinic was on one of the floors of a four-story building. I had spotted the staircase and at once knew what I was supposed to do. I knew that I was supposed to climb them up and down, as I usually did at home or at the railway stations. "But what is this? Why are they pulling me inside one of those rooms, which is the doctor's waiting room, before I can climb to the top?"

I resisted because I did not wish to go in. I wished to climb up and down the staircases as I thought and was sure that I was supposed to. I resisted by pulling myself backward. "I do not need to go inside before I finish my climbing."

I was puzzled. Mother had never stopped me from climbing any staircase before. So why was she pulling me away from them now? I had no idea about what "doctor's appointment times" were then. And when I got puzzled, I got disoriented. And when I got disoriented, I got scared. I felt as if my whole existence depended on those staircases. "What if I stop existing when I stop climbing them?"

Panic took over my eyes, blinding them shut. It took over

my ears, deafening me with the sound of a scream, which was my own, as I recognized it. My existence became the sound of that scream. And as I heard that sound, I could not see anything anymore, not those staircases, not even the door through which I was supposed to go inside the doctor's waiting room. My body and my surroundings were dissolved in the sound generated by my scream. Once it took control, I knew no one had any power to stop it. I had no power to stop it either.

"Why don't you take the boy somewhere else?" The color of my scream had the bubbles of somebody's voice in it.

"Yes, why don't you take the boy somewhere else. We are getting a headache listening to him."

There were more bubbles in the matrix of the stretching color of my scream. While I saw everything around dissolve in my scream, I waited to see more bubbles of voices in its color. But I did not have to wait long.

The doctor came out to find out what the matter was. And who knows what he saw or what he thought? For he offered to see me before anyone else. And who knows what he saw in me? For he declared that I had cerebral palsy.

I was surprised that I could hear his voice clearer than any bubble. And thus I realized that perhaps I had stopped screaming. Otherwise, why did I not see the stretching color of my scream anymore?

Now I found out from the doctor's voice that I had cerebral palsy, which was why I screamed and the reason my voice could scream but not talk. I was prescribed some medication.

Those Building Blocks

I remember those building blocks scattered on the floor. They had all those colors of blue, orange, yellow, and red. I remember Mother teaching me how to build my own staircases with them. She added cubes and cuboids to every piece to build it higher and higher.

"Now which piece should I add?" she would ask me. I would hand her some piece.

"Well, I am sure that blue piece would look fine here. But how about finding me a red one?"

Sometimes I would get puzzled when she asked me to give her a specific color. For identifying a color as red was very different from handing her the red block after sorting it out.

A new task of sorting needed to be thought, planned, and acted according to the plan. The task of sorting out the blocks was very different from the passive interactions with colors and shadows within my mind. It required using my body in the right way, using the right organs of my body, and picking the right object by eliminating other distractions.

It was embarrassing for me if I did not get it right. No one wants to do something and then realize they did it wrong. However, it is better to be wrong at home than in front of one of those clinical psychologists who assess your intelligence not by what you think but what you can do. Mother was helping me to do the task in the right way, so that for my next psychologist visit I could perform something with blocks when they were presented in front of me so that she may not write "non-response" again.

This is how we began. Puzzles need to be solved. My difficulty needed to be settled. We first sorted out all the blocks by color. Blue ones went in a separate bowl. Yellow ones in a separate one, while orange and red ones too were separated. At first this task looked difficult, like every new task. I have heard many children and adults facing similar problems, and caregivers or parents explaining that it is either a "motor-control problem" or a "hand-eye coordination problem." Mother and I did not know such terms. For us the approach was, "Problem? Let's solve it together."

The task of sorting out blocks according to color was difficult for me. But since Mother and I both did the work together, which meant that both of us were holding the same piece while we did the sorting, I was soon familiar with the activity and understood what my hands were supposed to do. And as I grew more comfortable with the task, I could do it independently. Mother put no pressure on me, but I was impatient to see the building process of the staircases because

I knew that it would not be built till the colored blocks were sorted out completely.

It worked fine with me. I was thankful to Mother when, instead of asking my nervous hands to do the sorting all by themselves, she took my hands and helped me pick the blocks till I was confident with my hands. For I never can learn anything under stress. We built them and unbuilt them. We did it over and over again.

I No Longer Need to Climb

One day I realized that I did not have the urge to climb real staircases anymore. For I could build my own staircases. I also learned to build a pillar with those blocks, so that the staircase could lean against it. Mother made vegetables climb up them. Potatoes and okras and beans took turns to climb up the block staircases until a jealous cabbage rolled from behind Mother and brought down everything, breaking the pillar and staircase into a pile of block pieces and scattered vegetables. Mother scolded the cabbage every time the destruction happened.

"Some people get so jealous," she would explain to me, as we would start building the staircase again. "Next time the cabbage gets jealous, I am going to cook it and no one is going to stop me," she warned, looking at the cabbage.

We would build the staircases over and over again. Mother would make the vegetables climb up. Again and again the cabbage would roll from Mother's hands and destroy the zone of play.

"This time the cabbage is really getting cooked," Mother would announce and head toward the kitchen. I loved eating cabbages.

Escalator Ride

Many years later, when I visited London, I had my first escalator ride. Every tube rail station had them. I was fascinated. They interested me more than the trains. I wished to ride them over and over again. However, since I was older, my impulses were more under my control. Did I realize that three years from then, I would live on Hollywood Boulevard, with escalators in every metro station and every mall? A whole choice of escalators waiting for me. I could either go to Hollywood Highland metro station or I could go to the Chinese Theater. I might ride one in the Hollywood Vine metro station, or I could go to the Beverly Mall.

Some days I would wish to ride on all of them just to "have a feel," as I explained to Mother. She said that it was more my obsession than "having a feel." Then the escal⸗ ride became more than "just a feel." It became a necessit⸗ brushing my teeth.

I would ride the metro trains after school with ⸗ Arnel, every day, until Mother came back from ⸗ sometimes I would wake up in the middle of the n⸗ dering about them, missing them till I felt a chok⸗ tion. Then I would wake Mother, and urge her t⸗

me to the Hollywood Highland station for an escalator ride.

Since I could not handle the wild wave of my obsession, I had to take Risperidal, a neuroleptic drug, which helped me through my extreme obsessive stages. Those extreme obsessions happened like a sudden summer storm, with its rushing energy flowing within my body and mind. They happened with no definite direction and with a high and powerful intensity, ready to take control of my reason and behavior.

They paralyzed all my
Other thoughts,
So definite were they,
They had them absorbed,
They left havoc
Along their way,
They engulfed the nights,
And the stretch of days.
I heard banging of doors
From my own twisted hands,
Shadows screaming with worry,
Fear or confused triumph,
They powered me up
With a prolonged pain,
With no eyes to see,

No ears to listen.
They left me no mind
To think or realize,
They did their dance
Of some dreamless delight.

To think about it now, as I am sitting in my Austin home, I am thankful that I am away from those escalators. I can still sense my body ride one of them. I can sense their gentle vibration on my body as I cling to the handle, concentrating on the oblique climb upward or downward, ambitious to climb up once again. I thank my new situation because I am far from that engulfing obsession.

In fact, I happened to ride up escalators at the airport only last month, when I took a trip to one of the Florida beaches. I was surprised that they did not charm me much. I was more than surprised. I was relieved.

I must confess that I certainly miss some aspects of Hollywood, just as I miss India. But I know that to miss something is a way of growing up, and I will always look back on those memories, as I move forward with my body and mind toward self-improvement.

My work never progressed much in Hollywood because my mind was overstimulated. I could not concentrate on my writing because all my senses were drawn toward the outdoor attractions and experiences. I did some writing, but I would put it in the B-grade category.

My story of staircases and escalators may emerge again from some corner in my life, like a rumble from a dormant volcano now and then, perhaps never. But for now, I have said it all.

The Power to Control
Darkness and Light

Thomas Edison invented the most marvelous device of all
time, the electric lightbulb. I marvel at those bulbs, and I marvel at electric fans. I marvel at the sound of a song from a
radio for my ears to appreciate. And then I marvel at the electric switch, which has the authority over them all, to control
the environment with instant brightness and darkness. Once I
realized the power of a switch, I knew what I was supposed
to do. My hands would wait for any opportunity to turn
switches on or off whenever I could get a hold of them.

Since I was very small, perhaps two or three years old,
many around me thought that switches were a dangerous
thing for my hands to play with. One day I watched electri-
cians come to our house and move all the switches out of my
reach because people were scared that I might get a shock. I
had to be patient. I had to be very patient. I needed to wait
for the next opportunity to get my hands on one of the many
switches in the world.

Switches could be anywhere in the world. In a neighbor's
house. At a doctor's clinic. In Grandmother's house. In any-

body's house that my parents visited, and no electrician had worked to move them out of my reach.

I knew exactly what I was supposed to do with switches the moment people got distracted. I would turn them on and turn them off. At first, I turned the switches on and off slowly. Then it would get faster and faster, like the blink of an eye, as if the room was blinking at the chairs and other furniture, as if the furniture blinked at the walls. It all depended on what you were looking at, to see what blinked at what.

The lightbulbs were the best appliances to react to switches. They made the room bright or dark, moment to moment. As I did my work with the switches, it gave me a feeling of great triumph, as if I was holding the reins of those bright or dark moments in my hands. And those moments comforted me by their predictability. They could either be bright or dark.

Otherwise, moments could get out of control, when they became unpredictable and too large for my senses to accumulate all that they involved within their field. One moment, you may look at a picture, and at the same time you are aware of the pink wall around the picture, you are also aware of Jack's voice explaining something about the picture. The very next moment you are looking at the reflection through its glass frame, which is competing for attention while you are looking at the picture. You may see a part of the room reflected in the glass, and you may be so absorbed in the reflection that you may not hear anything more from Jack's voice because you suddenly discover that those reflections are conspiring to tell you a story. Jack's voice may float in that story as big or small bubbles.

Moments are defined by what your senses are compelled to attend to. A moment may include a shadow of Jack's chair falling on the floor or a pen peeping out from the pile of papers, perhaps wishing to have a voice so that it could say aloud, "Here I am! Here I am!" And within the same moment, there may be a sudden sound of laughter that can dissolve the stories told by the reflections and the sullen silence of the chair's shadow within its demanding noise, making you wonder which part of the funny story from Jack's voice you missed listening to while you were watching the giant blades of the fan pushing out every story and sound away from it with air.

Since moment to moment this or that could be so unpredictable, when my senses juggled with much more intensity and frequency, it was better to work with switches, turning them on or off in order to bring more predictability to my understanding and comprehension of my environment. Otherwise, it could get too fragmented and difficult to collect all the pieces and combine them into a complete picture of a real environment. And why should comprehending the environment become less fragmented if I turned the switches on or off?

The simple answer: I would overlook the pink walls around Jack's picture, overlook the reflection through its glass, overlook the shadows of the chair, and perhaps overlook the blades of the fan because I would just see one aspect of the environment. The illuminating aspect, with a controlled probability of either bright or dark. After controlling my visual senses, I would be able to hear Jack's story in greater detail because switching the light on or off would calm me. It would allow me to eliminate other visual distractions like shadows, reflections, and the movement of the blades of the fan.

And while Jack described his picture, would I wish to look at it? I do not think so. The story behind an object is far more important to me than the object. That is why a description of a situation becomes more important to me than the situation itself.

Mother would not allow me to push the electrical switches on and off in the neighbor's house. First, she would try to divert my attention toward some boring object like a spoon. "Now let's see how this spoon reflects our faces. Now let's see how these spoons fight." She would have a pretend swordfight with two spoons. Her left hand would hold one spoon, and her right hand would hold the second spoon. Then Mother would make war sounds of all sorts, sometimes attacking sounds, sometimes defensive sounds, or sometimes the fading sound of an injured soldier. I would wait for her to get tired, then I would return to those switches. The hostess of the house we were visiting would also wait for Mother to finish her spoon fight before going back to her own narration about a wedding she had attended.

"What is the use of going to someone's house, if I cannot carry a conversation because I am constantly trying to keep Tito from playing with switches?" Mother decided to stop visiting neighbors or attend any social gatherings.

"So what should I tell them about your not coming with me?" my father wanted to know.

"Can't you tell them that your wife is sick, down with a cold, headache, ankle sprain, or anything that can prevent one from walking?" Mother would suggest.

I would remain at home with Mother. What kitchen crockery would come out next in the drawing room, where we played? I wondered. Steel bowls would come out, and I know that she would arrange them by inverting them first. Next, she would arrange them into a pyramid, one bowl on top of two bowls. She would accept my help now and then, allowing one bowl to roll away so that I could fetch it for her.

Unpredictability

Often in this world, things do not work according to expectations. And when that happens, it can lead to a bigger disappointment. Disappointment can grow in a direction called frustration. Frustration happened to me around switches. It happened when, sometimes to my horror, the power would go out and the lights would not turn on or off, even at the command of the switches.

I would pull Mother to those switches and nudge her to turn them on. Neither the lights nor the fan would work. The complicated concept of a power outage was not something I wanted to listen to or understand, although Mother tried to explain it to me.

"What do power outages have to do with switches and lights anyway?" I would wonder. Wonder was all I could do because I could not talk. I could not even communicate through writing or spelling by pointing then. I would pull Mother back to the switches, so that she could make them work. I believed Mother could make anything happen.

"Sorry, there is no power," Mother would tell me, turning the switches on and off again.

I would pull her back to the switches. My trust in her

and the switches would fall apart if the lights did not turn on.

Mother and the switch — I was sure — were in a conspiracy to make me feel suffocated. My trust in the predictability of those switches would turn into a feeling of suffocation and then into fear. Mother, sensing my state of panic, tried to make a ding-dong sound with her voice, explaining to me that "switches made that kind of ding-dong sound when they faced power outages," as if I would believe that! She even tried to make a nasal ding-dong sound, as if to prove that it was not her voice but the voice of the switch that was making the sound. She tried to start a dialogue with the switch, asking the switch in her natural voice, "Mr. Switch, hello Mr. Switch, is that your voice making the ding-dong?"

Then she would answer in that nasal voice, which she wanted me to understand as the voice of the switch, "Yes, it is me, the switch, making that sound."

Her real voice would continue, "So, Mr. Switch, why are you making that sound?"

She would answer, being a fake ventriloquist, in that nasal voice again, "Yes, I make that sound when the power goes."

Then she would try and turn toward me in her regular voice with a "See, I told you that before!" while I would feel an explosion inside me.

"What makes her believe that switches talk when the

mirror cannot, when shadows cannot, when I cannot?" I was furious.

I can now understand her trying so hard to prevent a temper tantrum. However, I would hear a scream from my voice exploding all my disbelief, frustration, and anger anyway. And how long would that scream last? I do not remember because once my scream started, I would lose all control of my voice. No one had control over my screaming voice when the power would go; sometimes not even Mother's song could stop it. I am told that I would stop only if I was exhausted, or if the power was restored.

Finally, I made a rule in the house. The fans in the rooms had to be turned on wherever I went. In that way, I could keep an eye on the power, believing that it would not go out if I kept an eye on it. And the fans would let me know whether or not the power was there. I did not play with light switches anymore, for now my fancy had moved toward ceiling fans.

The Power of a Ceiling Fan to Make Me Feel Sure

India is a tropical country. Most of the year, ceiling fans are needed. Air conditioners are there, but can be afforded by just a handful of people. So most of us have to rely on ceiling fans to provide us with some relief during the months of March to September. And what a relief it was for me to watch the ceiling fans rotating in every room of the house!

Heat made my body feel sick. I could not bear heat. The breeze, which the fans circulated, comforted my body and brought peace of mind. Just to know that the power was there gave me some peace. As my body felt secure and comfortable, I could think clearly.

I got attached to the ceiling fan day by day. Soon I began to depend on it. I would watch the opaque blades move faster and faster, as the fan would pick up acceleration, and then become transparent in the color of air, so that the ceiling could be seen clearly. Then it would look like a transparent circle, moving below the ceiling.

I would wonder about where the positions of its blades could be, as the fan moved. I would stand right below it, and rotate my body as fast as I could, wondering whether I too became as transparent as the fan. It felt wonderful to think that way. I could gather my body parts while I rotated, so that I could feel my arms, legs, and fingers, in total control. And what did I see while I rotated, competing with the fan's blades?

I could see a very blurred world, racing around me in the other direction. Once again, I felt sure of my movements and what I was supposed to see as I went around at that speed. Feeling sure calmed my senses.

The hunger to feel sure increased within me, so that I wanted to feel sure all the time. I went from room to room, in order to rotate my body under the ceiling fans, intoxicated with feeling sure. Sometimes I heard my own laughter emerging from myself, and being thrown out in all directions like a big spill of sound.

While I got intoxicated in that feeling, for most of my day, especially when Mother was busy in the kitchen, I began to miss out on a bigger part, which my environment had to offer me. I began to miss out on the richness of the surroundings because, when I rotated at that speed, like an addiction victim, my thoughts were too focused in the kinesthetic sensation of my movement. The sense of rotation, speed, direction, trying to remain below the fan, belief of becoming transparent like its blades, and losing my other thoughts, other than being in a state of total happiness, kept my heart occupied. I missed out on the sights and sounds of my environment. I missed out on the thoughts of shadows, thoughts of staircases, or thoughts of the stories forming and dissolving behind the mirror.

There were the ebbs and rise of sounds and sights.
There were voices of people, and sounds of day.
There were shadows on walls, otherwise filled with light.
I was nowhere near them, for I was far, far away.
Mother would enter the room from somewhere.
She would turn the switch of the fans off.
I would watch the blades of the fans turn slow and slower.
Till they would come to a dead stop.

I would stop rotating once the fans stopped rotating. But if the fans stopped, we would both feel hot. I knew for sure that Mother would be bound to turn them on again after fifteen or twenty minutes. Surely I could wait that long. I would wait, keeping my nerves alert. And I waited till it got too hot inside the room. And when it got very hot, she switched on the fans once again.

She would not let me rotate under the fan once she was in the room with me. In order to stop me, she began to place a table or a chair underneath it. Sometimes she sat right under the fan, knowing very well that I would not be able to rotate anywhere else, with her "Now what will you do?" face.

I would, however, try to rotate in a different corner of the room, with my "I can still do it" face, but it did not feel the same as rotating below the fan.

"Why do we need to be in that corner and feel hot when this book is waiting for us with all its pictures?" Mother would invite me to look at a book. But this is the story of the fan. So I will not include picture books in it.

Power Outages Happened, Despite the Moving Fan

The fan became my messenger, letting me know when the power went. I felt sorry to see that it could not stop the power outages.

When there were power cuts, I felt helpless and scattered once again, as if my existence depended on the movements of the fan. I would try not to worry, as I had learned from my early experiences that these were temporary situations. However, wishing away a worry is not the same as a worry actually going. And trying not to worry is not always enough.

So what would I do? I would try at first not to look at the fan, but I would still look, just in case. . . . Then I would try harder not to look at the fan, but I would still look anyway, getting upset with either my temptation, or my eyes, or the blades of the fan. "When will they restore the power?" I would wonder.

Mother would sense my anxiety, and try to distract me by reading or turning the pages of one of the books fast, which I began to enjoy under the moving fan. We could not go outside in the baking heat of the summer noon in India, when even the skin of one's body wants to melt away.

I would sometimes try to flap away the anxiety with my hands, getting worried and thinking of nothing else but the halted blades of the ceiling fan. Mother would sometimes call the local power station to check when they would restore power, so that I would not have another panic attack. I would feel my anger in my blood, waiting to be pushed out by a big breath from my lungs. I could see nothing else after that. Nor could I hear anything. I was surrounded by absolutely nothing. The surrounding was filled with the completeness of absolutely nothing, when such a breath waited inside my lungs. And then, into the color of nothingness, the color of my waiting scream would spread, like streaks and splashes, dissolving into the dampness of a heated summer noon.

Mother found a long pole one day. She kept it in the corner of the room, making me wonder what it was for. Then I knew . . .

One day, when there was another power outage, I knew why the pole was brought in. She stood in the middle of the floor, under the fan. And every time I got anxious about the power outage, she stroked one of the blades with that pole. That would make the blades take a turn or two. It kept my voice quiet.

The movements were slow. The blades would not be transparent because they would not attain the required speed. But it was still movement. I could at least feel the power of the pole, over the electric power. "Surely Mother can make anything happen!" My trust in Mother returned. I did not feel suffocated anymore.

Mother stood guard with her long pole under the fan during every power outage, keeping away my tantrum and my scream!

Power Outages Followed through My Older Years

My love for music and tape recorders started when the sound of the ceiling fan took the background, keeping its distance from my focused attention. It began between the ages of seven and eight. My ears got used to hearing music from tape recorders. The music kept me busy till I was ten years old.

When I started my eleventh year of life, I experienced changes in my hormones. I found a fresh rush of emotions flooding in when the ceiling fan stopped moving. I was surprised at this returning obsession. Mother was surprised, too. How could this trait of childhood obsession come back all over again after so many years? Didn't I boast about its extinction to people who asked me several questions about my extinct traits? But one thing I must confess all along. My body cannot tolerate heat. If I am hot, it takes up all my energy, and like a termite, it begins to eat up all my reasoning power.

Where was I when I was ten? Mother and I lived in a small two-room rental apartment in one of the market areas of Bangalore, India. Houses were close to each other. The sound of a door closing in one house could be heard by houses on either side of it. And the sounds of any day would be the sound of traffic on the main road outside the houses, the sound of the temple bell ringing across the street, the sound of a loudspeaker announcing the coming of a political leader, the sound of a vegetable vendor, the sound of women bargaining with a vendor from an open window, the sound of someone's television set, the sound of an infant crying along with the sound of street dogs arguing about some sensitive issue around an open garbage can. I mixed in that sound, the music from my tape recorder and the faint sound of the ceiling fan. I could not hear anything less.

The power would go in Bangalore, too. I would try not to be bothered, and yet be bothered. I would try to ignore its absence, yet not quite be able to accept its loss. So I would start pacing the small room with anxious steps. "Wonder how a caged tiger feels!" I would think about one of those tigers pacing inside a zoo cage.

Mother would try to talk in order to get me distracted. I would hear, yet I could not listen to her voice or to her words. She would allow me to have some space, by moving away to the other room. I would hear her lock the front door, so that I might not create some kind of scene outside and draw attention from the neighbors.

Then I would try to pace two rooms, because the limits of one room got too small to hold my anxiety. I felt sick, as I got tired of pacing. Mother would give me some biscuits to feed my nerves, more than my body. Then the body grew like a prison, trapping all the anxiety and heat within its own limits, melting away the mind, somewhere inside. There was nothing else I could do. I had stopped the habit of screaming now.

This time I heard a groan from my voice. I grabbed whatever I could like a drowning man. I grabbed Mother and realized that it was her hands, trying to get free from my clasp. I heard her voice, softly cautioning me that I might create an accident, if I did not think about what I was doing. I took a long breath and released her hands to find them red with pressure. And I began to fear my own self. I could not trust myself anymore. "Are you going to tell your friends about what I did?" I asked Mother. By then I could write and communicate. (I started writing and communicating when I was six. Speech was always difficult for me, and my speech cannot be understood by others. But I am told by encouraging friends that it is getting better. An encouraging lie is welcome, too. I politely thank them.)

I asked Mother whether she would tell her friends about my aggressive behavior by writing my words on a paper. I depended on paper and pencil to communicate my opinions and worries. My aggression and grabbing got more and more frequent as more and more power outages took place, and went past an hour. She replied that she was not sure whether telling someone would help things out or not. Perhaps it might go with the coming of the monsoons, when cities in India get cooler.

She was prepared to keep my aggression during power outages a secret, within the limits of the closed front doors of the two-room apartment, as long as I kept the sound of my groaning low. Otherwise, neighbors might hear me and wonder. She did not want the matter to be the principal topic of neighborhood gossip.

Monsoons came with the coming of June. It did bring a great relief to the city of Bangalore and also into our two-room apartment. Most electricity in India comes from a hydroelectric source. Hence, the monsoons brought overwhelming rains to the rivers and power outages became less frequent.

And what happened to the remaining part of my story about the fan? Nothing further . . . because I was invited that monsoon month of July to the United States, never again to be bothered by power outages and suffocating heat.

Stories — stories back and forth
Come again as memories swing.

Feeding My Body

My next story goes back in time to when I was six years old. That was the year I learned to eat all by myself. And that was the year I learned to dress all by myself, and be independent in the bathroom.

I did not know how to tackle a plate of rice, although I knew that it was my lunch. In India, normally people do not use forks or spoons to eat at home. Sometimes people are ridiculed by cousins if they see someone daring to use a spoon. "What happened to his hands?" they would ask.

I could not touch anything sticky. The experience of getting sticky rice on my hands made my nerves freeze. Yet I needed to learn how to eat rice with my hands because everyone is supposed to learn the traditional way of eating.

I could eat bread and dry food, but I would not touch rice. Someone needed to feed me rice till I was five.

I was seeing Prathibha Karanth, who was my mentor and a speech pathologist during that time. I called her Kaki. Kaki was the head of the department at the All India Institute of Speech and Hearing in Mysore, where Mother and I lived for three years before we moved to Bangalore. Kaki asked one of the student therapists, Shantala, to help me get used to eating sticky food, using my hands, as well as using a spoon.

I am thankful to my speech therapists in Mysore and Bangalore because they did not limit their work just to speech. Shantala asked Mother to bring my lunch to the institute every day. Mother was supposed to pack me rice, lentils, and vegetables, and carry it to the institute. Shantala dedicated her therapy time to work on my Indian-style rice-eating skill. She took my hands, without giving me any time to pull away my hands, and dipped them into the sticky mixture of rice, lentils, and vegetables.

My hands, as I can still remember it, felt too surprised and I saw them stick to the plate. Shantala tapped my knuckles as a reminder, so that I would pick up the food and eat. Bit by bit she helped me by taking my hands in and out of the sticky food on the plate, and then in and out of my mouth, tapping her reminders along my arm, knuckles, and elbows every time they froze. The whole process of that day's lunch took a long time to finish. I am not sure how long it took.

Shantala helped me to desensitize my tactile defense against rice during lunch every day. Mother continued to desensitize my tactile defense against it at home. By the end of one week, I had gotten used to the Indian way of eating rice. Now no cousin would want to know what happened to my hands. And no relative would comment anymore that Mother was spoiling me by feeding me rice.

Holding a spoon was another circus for me. I would hold the spoon, try picking up the food, and by the time it reached my mouth, things would spill out. Did I really care? I do not think so.

Mother asked Shantala to help me learn that, too. Shantala held the spoon, along with me, helped me pick up the food, and most important of all, saw that it stayed on the spoon till it reached my mouth. She allowed me to take my time eating, but saw that I completed the work.

At first, I could not make eye contact with any task that-was new. So I could not look at the plate or what the spoon picked up. Wherever the spoon landed, I scooped that part up. But as my hands grew familiar with the task, I began to look at what I was picking up. Looking at the task while doing it speeds up the process of learning any skill for me. And with speed, motivation grows.

I got ambitious with my spoonwork, as I became more determined to put the food in my mouth without letting it spill, choosing what to pick up first.

"Wish He Could Dress Himself"

"What else do you want Tito to learn?" Kaki asked Mother.

"Wish he could dress himself, without needing my help." Mother told Kaki that I was six, and she would not want to help me with my shirts and pants when I grew bigger.

"He can put on his underwear and pants," Mother assured Kaki, for I could sit on a stool, put my legs in, then pull the underwear or the pants up. If I did not sit on a stool, I lost my balance.

Shantala helped me learn how to wear my T-shirt. I learned to judge which was the front and which was the back of the shirt from the tag. She helped me by getting half my head in, so that I could pull my head out. It was uncomfortable to remain in a shirt that blocked my view. Then she put my hands inside the sleeves. I could push out my arms. It did not feel comfortable to keep my hands tucked halfway through the sleeves.

Getting the shirt off my body was easier. Shantala pulled my arm halfway out of one sleeve. The mere feeling of discomfort made me pull that arm out completely. Then the feeling of the stretched shirt, with one hand free of a sleeve, was no comfort either. I had to struggle my way out of it.

Shantala rewarded my attempts with a game of Memory, a game where picture cards needed to be matched to identical picture cards. I loved it because Shantala would allow me to win all the time.

As I worked with my shirt at the institute five times every day, I got used to the movements required through the muscle memory of my hands. Shantala needed to help me less and less after about two weeks with the shirt. My confidence grew with practice. Mother helped me practice wearing my shirt at home, too. Now I could put on my shirt — any T-shirt — all by myself after my bath.

Next, Shantala helped me learn how to wear a regular shirt with buttons. Shantala put my arm in one of the sleeves for me at first. She brought the other sleeve around my back, within my reach, so that I could put my other arm in easily. Next, we did the buttons. She put three-fourths of each button inside the hole. All I had to do was pull the rest of it out of the buttonhole. To button my shirt, I used only one hand at first. I could not use two hands in two different ways.

Buttoning needs two hands working in two different ways, each hand supporting the other in a cooperative effort. But the use of both my hands at first was not wise. I wore and unwore the shirt five times, working one arm and hand at a time at first. As Shantala began slowly to put more responsibility on me with my shirt, without realizing it, I soon started using both my arms and hands. Once I understood the task, I could map it well around my body. Every successive try got this kind of mapping well established in my mind. I could do the sleeves independently. Shantala sometimes helped to pull it around my back, left side to right side. And I began to map out the buttons, not just like a visually impaired person, as I previously did.

I wore my shirt in the beginning like a visually impaired person because I could not look at any new task. I learned to look at them as I got used to them. Later, I worked the buttons in and out of those buttonholes by looking at them.

A skill is learned faster when my eyes see them. Wearing a regular shirt became easier once my eyes dared to look at what my hands did. Mother and I practiced the activity at home. By the end of a month, I could dress all by myself.

Was I proud of myself after learning how to dress? I do not remember being proud. But I remember being relieved, and feeling like a grown-up. The process of learning this skill was too gradual for me to feel a sudden sense of pride.

When Learning Turns to Obsession

One day, I gave Mother a surprise. I removed my shirt at a bus stop, only to re-wear it, while she was looking in the other direction! When she turned and looked at me, realizing what I was doing, it was already too late. I was putting it on again. From then on, Mother placed me where she could see me. Once she even put safety pins on the shirt, just in case.

One lazy summer morning, when Mother went downstairs to fetch her usual bucket of water for cooking and drinking, I got very busy, trying on and taking off all my shirts till the last one. When she entered, I was standing in the midst of a heap of shirts!

It was fun to grow up and get new shirts from everyone. Since I could communicate, I was asked what color I preferred. I would specify my choice of stripes or checks or some color, whichever my mood commanded me to write.

The fun part of new shirts in India was visiting the men's tailors. They can be found on any corner. The tailor would measure me first. He would give an estimate of the amount of cloth he would need to stitch me a shirt. I felt like a very important person. Then we would go to one of the many fabric stores, where the salespeople would unroll all those shirt pieces in a heaped display, leaving me very puzzled as to which to leave and which to choose. Finally, I would decide because the salesman would bring another pile of shirt-roll fabrics from which to choose. He would perhaps say that they were the latest designs "now popular in Bombay," just to make me feel as lucky as someone wearing the same shirt walking on one of the streets of Bombay.

The salesman would not leave me till he succeeded in making me choose one. "No, no . . . You do not need to go to the next fabric store when our store has everything! And this lilac-and-blue check, wasn't it made just for you?" He would explain why I needed to choose the lilac-and-blue check; "Otherwise, your shopping would be incomplete, like a violin without its strings, the moon without the sky, the sea without salt. . . ." He would grin at his persuasive power if I finally decided to take two yards of one of his pieces, to appreciate his efforts at least.

I admired those salesmen in India, listening to their words and sense of humor and how they created a relation-ship with their customers. They would present every item, with such background talk that before leaving the store with that shirt on your back, you would appreciate every cotton farmer, every textile mill worker, and the textile designer who had worked on that fabric.

I miss those fabric stores in the United States. I see shirts, ready-made, hung in the clothes stores, with a "buy it if you want" or "don't buy it if you don't want" attitude, with no salesmen but tags to guide you. I feel that although I am in a very advanced country, with a comfortable life, perhaps I miss certain things about India.

Do I regret it? No, I do not. Perhaps salesmen are better suited to one environment than another. Just like sugar goes with ice cream but not with pizza. And I love them both.

The Torn Shirts

Eight years later, while I was in Hollywood, I ripped off my shirt during a temper tantrum, which began in one of the special schools for autism in Sherman Oaks, California.

The experience of school was new to me. I had not been accepted to Indian schools before. Mother was always my school. She taught me science, math, geometry, and poetry appreciation, along with other necessary subjects.

"If you really want to write," she would explain, "you must know everything from science to history to politics to religion." So she read Spinoza and Plato's *Republic* to me. I got lessons in coordinate geometry, as well as history.

Once I came to California, I had to go to school because Mother had to work in the mornings, so that we could continue to stay in the United States. Although the school program was a chaotic one, which was aimed more at the behavior development aspect than the cognitive aspect, I had to tolerate being there.

"Why can't we go back to India?" I asked Mother.

"In India," she explained, "we would need to wait a century for autism to be considered a disability. Here in the United States, there will be some care for you after I die." To ensure that, she needed to earn enough for us, that is, herself and me.

I understood her concerns. Yet I did not understand why I needed to be in a school.

"School is a structured place, and it is better than roaming around on the streets. Moreover, it would be less expensive for me if you went to school because I have to hire someone to be with you when I work." Mother gave me these two reasons for going to school.

The streets of Los Angeles were different from Indian streets. I enjoyed the metro rides and the downtown pavements. Being in school meant not being able to go downtown.

There was another reason for my disliking school. Art projects. Teachers did not really know what to do with me throughout my day. So they gave me markers and papers and crayons and all that junk to make a Picasso out of me, if they wanted me to be one at all, or to try to keep me occupied.

I must admit that I cannot draw beyond stick figures. Every time I tried drawing something, I would get so embarrassed. I had no mental model or map in my mind, and did not really know what I was drawing. And when teachers tried to be dishonest about it by praising me with a "Good job," I was more humiliated. Do they not know that I have two books published and one translated into German?

Why didn't I tell them? The answer is not simple. I wish I could initiate my wishes more than I could initiate my impulses. I wish I could write and communicate in every circumstance, no matter what it is. But if I could do all that, I certainly would have something other than autism.

After hearing that annoying singsong "Good job!" I had a sudden gush of anger. I grabbed my own shirt by the collar, and ripped off all my buttons. My aide, Arnel, had to staple them back on for the rest of the day.

I had more rage attacks in school, and my shirts had the same destiny. I had one just before entering the classroom. I was standing at the head of the queue of students, who were all waiting to enter the classroom. The moment I opened the door, there was a most annoying chorus of "Good job!" not only from the teacher but from those half-educated teacher's assistants who don't even know who Byron or Shelley was, and who believe that every act of a student needed to be Amen-ed by a "Good job."

"What is such a good job about opening a door? Do I have cerebral palsy?" I wanted to scream at them. But wanting it is different from making it happen. So my next shirt buttons got ripped out early that morning. Arnel had to staple up this shirt, too. It was a favorite shirt of mine. And because it was one of my favorite shirts, Mother had to stitch back the buttons that evening. For a few months, Mother had to stitch back many more buttons till she got tired.

"Sorry, you have to wear just T-shirts now. I can't be stitching every day after coming back from work." Mother knew how I disliked wearing T-shirts. But she would not stitch any more buttons! Since she would not stitch buttons on my regular shirts, I found myself wearing those cheap T-shirts, with my arms exposed. The skin of my arms never felt comfortable so exposed, as they are more sensitive, so I prefer to keep them covered by long shirtsleeves.

"You can staple my shirts if you don't want to stitch those buttons back, like Arnel does," I suggested, in writing. Mother would do none of that because she wanted me to be rid of the habit of taking my anger out on my shirt.

After we moved to Austin from Los Angeles one and a half years ago, Mother's employer and friend, Linda Lange, gifted me some snap-button shirts, which had long sleeves. What a great comfort those shirts were, after so many months of wearing only T-shirts. I could never rip those snap-button shirts anymore, although once or twice, I pulled them apart. The buttons just opened, then when I was no longer angry, I snapped them back together.

Habits form and habits grow,
Then some time later, habits go.

I can now assure myself that I do not let my anger fall on any shirt. And to my surprise, I have not had such a bad rage attack in several months. I have yet to see. . . . And I will have no shame in writing about it.

Walking in My Shoes

Many years may pass in my life. And year by year, stories may gather. The story of my shirt may be included somewhere and add up to my shirt tales, which began, "Once upon a time, when I was around six, when a wonderful speech therapist called Shantala went beyond her job to help me learn the motor skills!"

There waits in my head a new story, the story of my shoes. It is a story about my adapting to new shoes. And it is the story about my learning how to put them on and tie the shoelaces.

Certain memories are too difficult to forget. When a memory is associated with some extreme sensory activity, it is often hard to forget.

"How can you remember things about such early days?" someone asked me.

"Blame it on my extreme sensory activities. It is the factor that led me to remember certain aspects of my early days, although I sometimes cannot remember who I met at the store just yesterday."

From my childhood photographs, I know that I wore some kind of blue cloth shoes as a baby. They were my first shoes. I know that I wore them when my feet were really small, and when I could not walk. Those photographs also tell me that I had, in fact, two kinds of blue shoes, both made of cloth.

Then I learned to walk. And I have a very distinct memory of leather shoes, which Mother got for me. They were white, and they made a squeaking sound the moment I stepped forward because of some kind of air gap, purposely created to make that sound. Why did I have them, out of all the shoes in the world? Mother thought they looked good, and they sounded cute.

I was terrified of them. New shoes made my feet look detached from the rest of me. My senses got so strained that I refused to lay my feet on the ground. I was not more than two years old then. And I remember it through the intensity of that experience, which accumulated my senses, all at once, merging together with banging stress. I refused to lay my feet on the ground. I refused to stand with those shoes on, although Mother was clapping her hands to encourage me.

Mother heard me scream, just as I heard my voice scream. And Mother allowed me to scream. Mother later told me, when we communicated, that she wanted to desensitize me from my fear. She did not know anything about autism then. We did not know why my senses revolted so strongly then. All I know is Mother assured me she would remove them after fifteen minutes. "You just tolerate it for fifteen minutes," I heard her through my pauses, while I screamed.

Many days passed, each with the fifteen-minute promise. I even began to believe that the end of fifteen minutes was some magical moment, when every sorrow, every fear, and every scream in the world ends.

And did I know then that Mother was extending her fifteen minutes by a longer and longer duration? I did not know the tricks Mother knew! So I began to come to a truce with my squeaking leather shoes. "After all, she removes them after fifteen minutes."

Those shoes turned out to be harmless, after all. I wore them all evening for a walk around the township, where we stayed, still believing that I wore them for just fifteen minutes.

One day I got another pair of shoes because my feet grew bigger in size, and those squeaking white shoes could no longer carry my growing feet. I panicked with every new pair, I am told. But the magic of fifteen minutes, and the assurance that after fifteen minutes, all the troubles of the world would end with the removal of my new shoes, kept my feet growing and kept my shoes witness to their stages of growth.

A long time ago it was.
And still alive in my mind.

As those shoes got worn out,
To leave them years behind.

Today, I am close to turning eighteen. Do I still fear wearing new shoes? My answer is no. I still feel uncomfortable and stiff with new shoes or slippers. But not to the extent that I would need to scream out my discomfort, as I once did, wishing it would scare those squeaking white leather shoes in which my feet felt and looked so different. I feel uncomfortable, yet I can endure.

A Grip on the Shoelaces

Mirror, mirror, on the wall,
Gather stories big and small.

I looked at the mirror today, as Mother was teaching me how
to shave, using a charged razor. I could see the mirror reflecting my six-year-old hands, learning how to tie shoelaces. It
was in the city of Mysore, in India, where I lived, where I
learned the skill of tying shoelaces.

We had a skipping rope at home. Mother and I used that
rope to tie around the armrest of the chair every day. Both our
hands held the rope, as Mother held my hand, to practice
tying the first knot around the armrest. We needed a thick
rope, so that I could feel it and hold it better. We practiced
knot-tying several times a day as a habit, morning and
evening, just like we had our habit of breakfast and dinner.
We practiced it every day. There was no pressure on me or on
Mother regarding learning time, so there was absolutely no
stress.

Mother bought many nylon ropes, which came in different colors to tie around the chair. We had yellow and green
and magenta, shocking pink, red, and black nylon strings. She

stood behind me because she wanted me to focus on the work, rather than on her. I am so glad that she never stressed me out with some demand like, "Look at my eyes." I heard her voice behind me speak, while we tied the knots together continuously, "I think this yellow knot would not want blue knot around it today. . . ." She continued with her soliloquy without caring whether or not I really believed her story.

"If you ask me why I think so, I would have to tell you that those two colors have quarreled today. And if you really want to know why I think they quarreled today, I may ask you to have a look at the sky. See, the yellow sun and blue sky are not looking at each other today because of those clouds. And be sure, those clouds are here to stay, at least for this day." Mother assured me not to worry much because colors usually make up any quarrel, as if I had any reason to worry why yellow and blue quarreled. But yet I worried and wondered.

I would continue to tie the ropes around the armrest, wondering what the mirror had to say about yellow and blue. I would look at those colored knots tied around the chair and wonder what interactions went on between them because Mother told me how shocking-pink rope and black rope were best friends that day.

Mother gave me many reasons why she put certain colors together, in case I wondered. And I did wonder.

She told me about all the possibilities that the colored

ropes could make, and that the mathematical calculations of permutation and combination could help us find that out. I, however, looked forward to my task of learning how to tie a knot because I wanted to hear her reason-stories. Knots of all colors came alive once they each had a character.

"Today this black knot wants to be very secure, so let's pull it tight. . . ."

In the beginning, Mother held the rope ends around my hands, guiding me through every movement. "We are making a letter O first, around the chair. . . . And now letter O wants to raise both its hands up . . . like this." She brought the two ends to my eye level. "Now these arms must fold, one has to go inside O . . . ," while we made the knot. "All we have to do now is pull them . . . like this."

As days passed, with the ritualistic tying of those colored nylon ropes, I got to map out the movements more clearly. My confidence in my motor movements improved. After some weeks, Mother pretended to get distracted, removing her hand from my hand, which held the rope all by itself, doing what motor memory had learned. If that "all by itself" arm froze, Mother held it again, so that I would not feel threatened. Sometimes the left hand, sometimes the right hand continued the task, as Mother pretended to get more and more distracted. Soon, I held the rope all by myself, first making the letter O around the armrest, raising the arms up, passing one hand inside the O, then pulling the arms apart. But I was no longer scared, for Mother always made me feel that she was there.

Both my hands knew how to tie the rope around the armrest. I learned how to make the second knot, too, in the same way. I had to repeat the same process by making rabbit ears with the rope. This took less time.

Then Mother replaced those thick nylon ropes with shoestrings. I had to begin the same way, tying the string around the armrest. I knew the movements . . .

> "Letter O around the chair,
> Raising up their hands,
> Passing one hand inside the O,
> And pulling them apart."

— I recited as I tied.

Finally, I graduated to real shoes, first without wearing them, just placing them on my lap. Once I could do that, I wore them, tied them up completely, to step ahead with independent walking feet.

> Stories restored step by step,
> To move my words somewhere ahead,

Stories long, stories short,
Never leave me, out of their stock.
So with my feet, stepped in shoes,
I stick to old shoes, but accept the new,
Strings get tied, every one,
I step along, I walk along.

"How Do You Perceive a Linear Situation?"

"How do you perceive?" I am asked many times. And since every question has an answer, other than the question, "Can God create a mountain which He cannot break?" the question asked to me certainly needs an answer. And answering a question is a social task, which I ought to do.

When I was five years old, and was just learning about my sense organs, I would have answered that question with, "I see with my eyes, I smell with my nose, I hear with my . . ."

As I grew up, I wondered many things. I learned the laws of reflection. According to which, a mirror is nothing but a plane surface made of a supercooled liquid called glass. But why does it become so alive to me? And why should any shadow have the power to stop stories from forming? Shadows are nothing other than unlit parts.

Do other people see things the way I do? I needed to study neuro-typical people, and how they perceived things, to understand the answer before answering people. So I asked Mother how she saw things. I was surprised by her answer.

She said that when she saw a book,
- she was aware of what I was doing;
- at the same time, wanting to make herself a cup of tea;
- and being uncomfortable at the thought that she was running out of rice, and next day at the latest, she would need
  to buy some;
- she could hear the fan and the sound of a passing car on
  the street;
- she could feel cold, and yet she could see the book.

Or when she cooked,
- she was aware of her environment;
- she was aware of the colors, smells, and temperature in the
  kitchen;
- she also wondered what I was doing because I wasn't
  around her;
- she would feel guilty for not attending to me, while she
  cooked;
- she would also hope to read me something from the news-
  paper, once she was done with her cooking;
- and the very next moment be irritated that her cooking
  was taking so long.

I began to see the difference between her perception and my
perception. When I enter a new room, which I am entering for

the first time, and look at a door, I recognize it as a door, only after a few stages. The first thing I see is its color. If I do not get into a deeper cogitation of its color by defining it as "yellow," and mentally lining up all the yellow things I know of, including one of my yellow tennis balls when I was seven years old, I move to the shape of the door. And if at all I lay my eyes on the door hinge, I might get distracted by the functions of levers. However, I pull my attention from there and wonder about the function of that yellow, large rectangular object, with levers of the first order, called a hinge.

Why is that yellow, large rectangular object with levers there? I mentally answer the question, "It has allowed me to come inside that room, and can be opened or closed. And what else can that be, other than a door." My labeling is complete. And I move on to the next object in the room to find its characteristics, then define and label that object.

Does this happen for all circumstances? No, when I am used to situations, and have labeled the objects included in that situation many times, I do not need to follow these steps. I can label the situations and objects on my first step. And so, practice, exposure, and experience with objects and around objects matter a great deal, in order to accommodate new situations.

If I am out in a garden, where there is a garden tap, and water is filling up a red bucket, which is a dynamic situation, changing, from instant to instant, I first notice the color of the bucket. I might easily get distracted by its redness, since it would remind me of how my hands bled when I had fallen from a swing, how I was so absorbed in that red that I had forgotten about my pain, and how that red resembled a hibiscus. . . .

I would then realize that I was hearing the sound of water, wondering why that sound reminded me of a drowning man's last blood flow, although I had never seen a drowning man in real life, let alone the flow of his blood, or whether any drowning man ever thinks about the state of his blood flow.

The bucket is filled up eventually, and I see water spilling from it. I understand the situation, waking from my branching thoughts, summing up the components into one conclusion, which is "water filling up a red bucket from a garden tap."

Perceiving a Nonlinear Situation, with Unpredictable Results

Most situations are not linear. They vary from moment to moment. Like a game of football.

I tried to watch a football game on television, which had moment-to-moment shifts in the situation. The situation was multidirectional and nonlinear. Anybody could be anywhere at any moment. Because anybody could be anywhere, there could be no predictable moment. Every moment became unique.

I sat through the game, determined to understand why Lloyd, who worked as my aide last summer, was so glued to the football match, while I struggled to follow it. I tried to put a whole amount of effort into getting moment-by-moment information and processing it in my mind. The players looked like tickle ants, scattered on the television screen.

"Do you know the rules of football?" someone may wonder.

"Certainly I do. Don't the players of each team try to shoot a goal? Same as rugby, but players here are armed with a helmet and guards," I would answer.

Mother once suggested to me "to follow the ball because

players follow the ball." But when players hold the ball and run, it becomes a big challenge for me to find out who has the ball. And then it all seems out of control, as I see colors moving on the screen like tickle ants. I continue to watch it with Lloyd, not as a game anymore but as "tickle ant moves."

"Man, you enjoy it, ha? Good, good, man!" said my aide, when I couldn't control a smile at a few tickle ants tumbling over each other. Wasn't he wise to choose the right channel for my entertainment?

Watching a game of tennis is far easier. There are just two or four players in their predictable spaces. The ball is in a predictable position, too, for it can be either on this side or that side of the court. And when I can predict, it is easier to attend.

I have attended autism conferences, where people with autism have announced that they have the same understanding and the same interpretation as neuro-typical people. It always made me wonder about their claim, because I do not. I either over-see, or I under-see the components of the environment.

Once, in Bangalore, I visited a house and sat on a comfortable sofa in the drawing room. People who knew of my love for magazines would keep magazines for me because I loved to turn and touch those smooth glossy pages. On that day, I was sniffing each page of every magazine. I was so absorbed in smelling the pages that I missed seeing the piano, framed photographs, and lace curtains. I realized their presence, long after we had left that room, as Mother discussed the visit aloud on our way home. "Did you see those pink roses on the lace curtains? Wonder who plays that piano in that house! And did you see the little picture in the silver frame? It is her son . . . some kind of lawyer now."

On our way home, far from that real drawing room, where I had sat sniffing the magazine pages, I began to actually "see" the room coming back alive in front of my eyes. I could smell every article described by Mother, lace curtains, piano, and silver-framed picture, like the pages of magazines.

In a Crowded Place

I remember the railway station ticket office in Bangalore, India. It was a huge hall with a very high ceiling and with many counters. Railway is the primary mode of transport in India. I loved the place. What was so interesting to me?

It was the huge amount of movement and energy inside that booking office hall. Every time I visited it, I got a little more familiar with that place. There was always a big crowd. Was I threatened by it? No, I was not. For it was an organized crowd. Some people would stand in long lines in front of each counter. Those lines stretched parallel to each other. People would come and people would go. Each had a name and identity.

But to me, they were just people.
I was one of them.
Some people would sit on those red and black polymer
chairs, which were placed all around the walls of that hall.
I was one of them.
Some would walk in and out of those big glass doors.
I was one of them.
Some would walk in the canteen at the far end of the hall.

I was one of them.

Some would order apple juice from a little stall.

I was one of them.

Some would go into the magazine stall and buy some
    magazines.

I was one of them.

The more I went to the ticket office, the more I got to "time"
my senses as the events took place, so that I could isolate each
happening from any other.

   Since I could now easily recognize the door as a door and
the wall as a wall because I saw them so often, and since I no
longer needed to stare at the design on the mosaic floor and
wait for Mother to narrate to me what went around on me
while I was staring hard at the floor till my eyes watered, I
could look around me. I could see the crowd and smell the
crowd. I could hear the crowd and feel it grow around me. I
could see and smell the crowded room all at the same time. I
heard pieces of conversations in different languages. I could
understand some languages, while others I could not. The
ones I could not made me wonder about their words. I
formed my own translations just by guessing.

   I was so fascinated by the sounds and energy of the ticket
office that I began to visit it every week and then demanded to
go there every day. I was obsessed about visiting it. It became

like my pilgrimage, be it monsoon, be it summer, to visit it.

I had a big tantrum when Mother did not take me there one day because she thought that it was overstimulating me and my senses. I had begun to visit every shop and stall around it, so that we could do some buying. Mother called it "unnecessary buying" because we did not really need anything for the house.

"Why not? Don't I get to sit on those side chairs, with other people? Don't I get new magazines each time I visit?"

"But what about this plastic comb, which you insisted on buying from that roaming vendor. And what about that whistle, which you made me buy and lost all interest in once we got home? And this magazine! *Business India!* Do we need it? Why should we have it?" Mother was very careful with her money when we were in Bangalore. And each of my visits was a little more out of her planned budget.

My story of the railway station ticket office shows how my perception got used to a large area slowly. As I grew comfortable with it, I began to enjoy it. As I enjoyed it, I got addicted to it. And once I was addicted to it, I began to need it.

On a Swing

And all of that was left behind,
As with the graph of linear time,
I stood on a land so far from it,
And think of it with a longing mind.

I was allowed to use the campus of the Spastic Society of
Karnataka in Bangalore, although I did not go to school there.
They allowed me to be there so that I could socialize with the
students.

The campus had a swing. I spent most of my hours on
that campus sitting on that swing. What was my perception
from that swing? I don't think I paid any attention to my
vision when I sat there. Moving to and fro became the primary attraction, rather than what I should be seeing.

I sat there to hear the wind and feel the wind on my
face. It made me happy. It made me so happy that I became
addicted to it, a kind of pleasant addiction. I would go to the
Spastic Society building, and instead of going to any of those
classrooms, where I was supposed to socialize, I would run to
the swing. As if that was where I was meant to be.

I would sit on that swing, and rock my back and legs as

the amplitude of the swing increased. Mother would try to teach me while I sat on the swing. She would make my joyous experience a science class with a whole lot of whats and whys. Before coming to the Spastic Society campus, she would go through a lesson on how Galileo Galilee discovered the relationship between the duration of the oscillation and the weight of the pendulum bob. I was the pendulum bob of the swing. Mother would go through the relationship between the duration and the length of the swing and how Sir Issac Newton explained it all.

I would sit on the swing with a head full of scientific concepts and ears filled with the sound of the wind. My heart would be filled with happiness as it expanded or contracted, perhaps to the rhythm of the swing.

What exactly did I perceive while I sat on the swing? I perceived happiness in the colors of the wind.

Perceiving Faces

"Who did you go out with?" Mother asked me one Saturday.

"Mr. Lloyd," I answered.

"No, it was not Mr. Lloyd. It was Mr. Clifton," she corrected me.

"If you say so, then it was Mr. Clifton." I did not disagree with her.

Mr. Lloyd was a big man, with a broad smile. Mr. Clifton was a big man, too, and had a big smile. I took one for the other.

In order to get a permanent impression of someone's face, I need some time. How much time? It depends on how much interaction that face, and the voice generating from the face, has with me. Mr. Clifton happened to be a quiet person.

I always recognize the face of the Mona Lisa because of her perpetual smile and her looks. I am not very sure whether her face would be so familiar to me if she happened to frown or laugh with an open mouth or perhaps turn her head to one side. I will have no trouble recognizing her face as long as she keeps her head still. Her face was something I read about and studied.

Why did I mix up Mr. Clifton with Mr. Lloyd? This was

not the first time I encountered this problem. Often, people have complained that I have ignored them, making them wonder why I was so impolite. I wonder, too. I wonder about my perception because I do not mean to be impolite to any of those people. A face map is a very difficult and complicated thing to decipher.

Each face comes with the usual positioning of eyes, nose, and mouth. Yet they are so different, with different contours of facial bones. When I look at diagrams of skeletons and at pictures of face bones in the pages of *National Geographic*, I do not see any difference between those face bones, although some may have belonged to the Incas, brought to light by curious archaeologists, who would never let any heathen bone rest in peace. Those skulls with their perpetual smiles all look alike, although I know very well that when they had muscles and skin around them, they looked different from each other. Had I been born during that Inca period, I would have had equal difficulty in determining which face belonged to the priest, if I encountered that face in three dimensions. For the face would still tease me, "Tell me whose face I am?"

During the early years of my life, I did not look at anyone's face, although I was aware of their presence. I did not look at any face because I could not. I felt threatened when I looked at them, for every face demanded the identification of a name.

To identify a face needed a very careful "looking back" to match that face with a past encounter with it. My encounter with that face could have been in a park a week back. At this moment, it could be in a room where I had to match that face to my previous experience in the park, where perhaps I was busy building a story with grass green and leaf green. There, in that previous environment, I heard voices, including the voice coming out from his face. Those voices, including his voice, became part of that story in grass green and leaf green, dissolving in and out of my breath, making me wish for a mirror.

So in a different situation in one of the rooms in our apartment in Bangalore, Mother announced that "Mr. Rao came to see you because he wants to talk to you." I had to wait for him to talk first because Mother continued to tell me, "Remember . . . we met him last Sunday at Cabbon Park when he said he wanted to do a story on you?"

I remembered the situation but I still had to wait to hear his voice, so that I could pull it out from the right place of my memory, which would be in the story of grass green and leaf green, when I missed having a mirror around. Only when I heard his voice did I remember the exact moment that Sunday at Cabbon Park. The face matched the voice in that story in grass green and leaf green.

I took my pencil and wrote in my notebook, "Hello Mr. Rao."

As I mentioned earlier, I was listening to Mother singing me a song when I realized that her voice was generated when her lips moved. All moving lips are parts of faces, as unique as their voices. My speech therapist, Deepa, had shown me the diagram of vocal cords, explaining to me how when they vibrate, we can hear our voices, as we ritualistically tried to vocalize the sounds, "a-a-a—a" and "o-o-o-o—o," during therapy sessions. The diagram of the vocal cords was flesh pink and white.

As I continued my interview with Mr. Rao, I could imagine his vocal cords vibrate as he asked me all those questions and as I wrote down all my answers for him. I could imagine the colors of grass green and leaf green floating around, slowly being replaced by the white and flesh pink of his vocal cords. I could see the page on which I wrote turn slowly to a flesh pink, while Mr. Rao spoke aloud. I was in the midst of all those colors, holding on to my pencil, lest it get lost in the viscous stretch of white and flesh pink, which had the power to dissolve the green. Mr. Rao's identification was the sound of his voice, vibrating in a pool of flesh pink and white, fading out of grass green and leaf green. The interview was complete, and it was added to the story as the concluding part of that which began in grass green and leaf green. When I retrieved it for this page, my words had the same essence of those greens, with the smell of grass and leaves.

Would I recognize Mr. Rao again, if he stood in front of me at some point in my life? I might not recognize him by his face, but I would surely recognize him if I heard his voice. Maybe a new color would be added to the pink and white when I met him next. Maybe a new essence would be added to those colors. Who knows what would happen if I met him again to continue that story?

Without those stories, recognizing and recalling a person or a situation is very difficult.

Everyday Faces

"Is it difficult to recall or recognize a person I see everyday?" I must say, "No." For me, those everyday faces become more like an essence and habit. I no longer need stories to preserve the incidents with those I encounter every day. For example, in the beginning, Deepa's presence was just the sound of her voice, which tasted like tamarind pickle. As days passed, her presence became a peacock blue, dipped in the taste of tamarind pickle. A month later, when I was more used to her, she began to take a more visible shape than the representation of colors and tastes. I began to feel confident enough to look at her more, as I could clearly see her perfect beautiful face, which I would feel honored to dream about, even though I am several years past my encounters with her and I am many thousand miles away in the United States. Thus remained the memory of her face. Thus remained the essence of her presence as a poem.

> She was sitting in the clouds,
> She was floating like the moon,
> She was sitting through the night,
> She was singing through the dark,

She was looking through time,
Yet so distant like the sky.
She filled my very thoughts,
In the heart of every dream,
She was blowing through time,
All my outs and ins,
She was distant as the moon,
She is distant like the sky.

Sometimes faces are stored in my memory as symbols. Every time I hear the voice of my teacher's face in Austin, I see her presence as a yellow bowl. Her face is represented as a yellow plastic bowl with a wide circumference.

Why on earth should it be yellow and not red or green or blue? Why on earth should it be plastic and not steel or copper or china? Why should it be a bowl and not a cup or a glass or a plate? I do not have any answers to those questions. All I can say is that it just happens to be a yellow plastic bowl with a wide circumference I see each time I hear her voice or recall my experiences with her.

A whole year has passed since I have heard and interacted with her. Yet the representation of her has not changed. I have mentally tried to put some tulips in that bowl, so that she may be represented as a yellow plastic bowl, wide circumference, with tulips in it, but I could not retain that picture.

Magazine Pictures

How do I remember and identify pictures in a magazine? Pictures in the album and in the pages of a magazine are different. They are smaller in size and they are in two dimensions. They do not change their angles from time to time, and their expressions are frozen the moment the photograph was taken. They are nonthreatening because they never demand, "Now that my face is here, I would like a social interaction with you."

I can see the face of the president of the United States anywhere on the pages of *Time* magazine and recognize who that face belongs to, whether he frowns, smiles, or doesn't smile. The picture would not generate any voice for me to attend to my auditory sense because my auditory sense is more powerful than my vision, and usually takes over in a dynamic situation filled with sound and sight. So I have more time to look at that face in the magazine.

And what about the face of a newsreader on television? The face of a newsreader is very nonthreatening. He never expects a dialogue with me. His speech is a monologue, full of information. He never pauses to wait for my opinion. Even if he waits for an opinion, he takes it from some expert and not me.

Hearing the news is the same as listening to someone read a story to me. So I can stare at his face and focus on my auditory channel without the interruption of social talk.

I passively look at his face and listen to his voice. As I listen, I can see the stories he tells either from Iraq or some dark coal mine. I see those stories, sometimes in vermilion or indigo, the richness depending upon the intensity of the stories. Sometimes they smell like vitriol and sometimes they smell like boiling starch in a pot of clay. And sometimes they have the essence of the twilight sky.

As I feel my worries for the trapped coal miners, I can smell the boiling starch, frothing on the brim of the clay pot, then spilling out with the smell of burning rice. My worries grow as the voice of the newsreader continues to say that the miners are still trapped. I smell burning rice spread all across the room as more starch spills out.

The news continues with sports coverage showing footage of basketball and football, with a very happy crowd of spectators and very fast-moving players. My body begins to itch as though tiny black tickle ants have been set free from a box. They can smell the burning rice from the spilling starch, and they rush around to find the source with a collective ant hunger. My worry now accumulates in and across my itching skin, as the voice of the newsreader comes from far away, like a blue floating balloon. I have no hold on it because it floats away, leaving me with itchy skin.

Perceptions differ from man to man
And perceptions differ from man to dog
I see, he sees, or it sees the same things,
And perceptions tell us what is what,
And thus through some eyes, a rose may bloom,
Not as a mere yellow-petaled flower,
For through his eye the blessed would see,
The image of the tender hands of its Maker.

Exposure Helps Shape Visual Perception

When my senses get used to a situation or a circumstance, the real image or picture starts forming. How well do those pictures form in my mind? It varies, depending on my exposure to the intensity or the frequency of that situation or circumstance. The more exposure, the better the visual image. If the exposure is not enough, it remains a symbol, like a sound, smell, color, taste, or some combination of two or more senses. I have to be satisfied with the abstract memory of that situation. It helps me remember my interactions with my environment.

Once, Bill Hirstein, who was one of the scientists who tested me when I first came to the United States, picked up a toy tiger and placed it before me.

"Tito, name this object."

I began to search all the names that were associated with that object, like *carnivore, stripe, ferocious, forest, hunt,* etc. All those names appeared in my mind except the word *tiger.* I was getting desperate. I was getting desperate because I felt trapped in the focal points of the waiting eyes of those scientists who were ready to prove "Who knows what." And I was trying my best, too, as I tried to untangle the web of all those terms that had collected around that toy tiger. I had to get the word they wanted. Finally, to my relief, I could solve the problem. I wrote down my answer. "A striped animal, which is not a zebra, is a TIGER." That was easy.

After showing me the tiger, they showed me many more things and I had to name them all to prove "Who knows what." I defined all those words to retrieve the names. For example, when I was shown a picture of a flower, I wrote, "a soft petaled part of a plant is a FLOWER." When a plastic toy elephant was shown to me, I wrote, "a very big animal, which evolved from a mammoth, is an ELEPHANT." I did the entire test of object identification by defining or describing the object through its appearance and properties to find its name.

This test was different from the test administered by Dr. Judith Gould at the National Autistic Society in England in 1999. I was given a term, and I had to choose the right picture that went with the term. Dr. Gould was reading the terms aloud and a page was shown to me, on which I had to choose out of four sketched pictures. I made no mistakes because the terms were spoken and the pictures were definitions in themselves. Although both tests were aimed at finding the right word or matching the right picture to the word presented, one was easier than the other. The problem of determining the right noun was identical to my face identification problem.

In his book *Descartes' Error*, Antonio Damasio talks about the "converging zones" in the brain, which oversee the recollection of nouns and interactions between different nouns, like *fan* and *air*, *bus* and *driver*. These converging zones are also responsible for storing the images of faces, in general and in particular. Like the faces of Tibetan monks and the face of the Dalai Lama. In his book Damasio mentions two types of converging zones, the lower converging zone and the higher converging zone. The lower converging zone is responsible for storing a general image of faces, with two eyes, a nose, and a mouth below the nose. The higher converging zone is responsible for storing images of one particular face and recalling that face at the right moment from some past experience.

After reading that, I made my own hypothesis. I might have trouble with the higher converging zone regions of my brain. That may lead me to find it difficult to recall a person's name based on his face, although I can recognize who he is from his voice or his personality traits, which are usually stored as a symbolic representation or combination of different sensory stories. That is my hypothesis.

When I Think of the Wind,
I Am the Wind

Stories grow and they always grow
Through the this and that
Moments pass, moments follow
And memories ever-last.

When someone asked me about my writing, I had once written down, "When I see or think about the wind, I am the wind."

I see flying leaves around me, as I hear a powerful wuthering noise, which can invite those dark pirate clouds to fly and fight each other for territorial expansion across the sky. Sometimes I am the wind blowing across the desert of the Sahara, gathering bowls of dust in order to build a huge crescent-shaped dune in the heart of nowhere for the stars of night to see. Sometimes I am the wind in the mountains, where the snow leopards roam in search of the blue mountain sheep.

How do I perceive that? I do not need to perceive that because I am that when I think of that. Alive and all-powerful.

I think of a wall,
I am a wall.
I was built to stand.

Vertical, all-
enduring
Holding
a roof, above my head.
Responsible,
For I mark the boundary
Between the inside
And the outside —

I am a wall
I was built to stand.

I am sometimes a wall
A desperate wall
Of a storm-beaten house.
I feel the force of the wind
I feel the force of water
They push me harder
and harder.
Till I can resist no more.
I hear myself break

With a terrible regret.
I hear my last prayer
For those who trusted
Me for years.
Whom I cannot save.

I was a wall.
I was built to stand.

Overperceiving and
Underperceiving

There are components in the environment that I never miss. For instance, once I was at a cinema in Mysore, India. I was fascinated by the ceiling pattern of that big hall. There were little squares and bounding them were big darker squares. I mentally started to draw a long chain of diagonals across those little squares.

I began drawing my mental diagonals, from one end of the cinema ceiling, and continued drawing them all the while I sat there. As if that was the reason for my visit. The lights in the hall were turned off till the intermission. It did not bother me. I could still see the ceiling, or thought that I was seeing it, and continued my task of drawing diagonals all across. The lights were turned off again after the intermission for the movie to resume. I continued drawing from left to right, then again from right to left on the next row as a chain of zigzags.

There are components in the environment that I can miss due to the overindulgence of one sense or an overindulgence toward one component of the environment to which my perception chooses to attend. That day, while my senses were caught in the activity of drawing diagonals across the ceiling, I missed the whole movie. I missed out on the sounds and the story the movie had to tell.

Did I regret it? Not at all. For at the end I was satisfied to cover the entire ceiling with diagonals. And not a single square was left out.

In a school in the city of Sherman Oaks, I sat a whole day in a classroom, planting mental nails all over the walls of that room. While I planted those mental nails, I kept a count of them. I knew that those nails never existed in real dimensions, but when I planted them I experienced their hardness and their blackened shine. They kept my mind busy the whole day, from morning till noon and again after lunch break, until it was time for me to leave. I mentally placed them very close to each other, as if they were a plate full of mustard seeds.

People walked in and out of the classroom many times. Perhaps I did, too. But I was not bothered. I was very busy, as my mind carefully fixed those nails close to each other, counting and concentrating on the task. I was determined to finish with at least one of the walls before I went home in the evening. How could I have time to think of any other thing? Quite a goal for a day!

I was in my visual sensory mode that day. A visual mode, which my mind made me see, not my eyes.

There were sounds around me. I did not hear them. Or I heard them but did not listen. In that school, there was no interesting auditory impulse to challenge my mental visual task and pull me away from it. No one read any interesting thing to the students. The sounds were verbal commands like, "Sit down" or "Look here," or basic talk.

> There was monotone all around me.
> There was the wandering power of my mind.
> There were patches of light and patches of shade.
> There was the grayness of a paused time.
> There were footsteps now, then, here, or there,
> As I planted my nails with an imagined hammer,
> Rap-tap, rap-tap, I planted those nails,
> To fill my day from corner to corner.

"I had a wonderful day at school," I told Mother when she asked.

"What did you do there?" Mother wanted to know.

"I planted nails!" I told her.

I waited for her to read me *Swann's Way*. After a whole day of visual work my ears were ready to hear Proust's work. And my mind's eyes were really very tired, concentrating on the placement of every nail. Planting mental nails and remembering the numbers and allotting a place to each nail needed a whole lot of staring at the wall.

Why Couldn't I Draw a Sun?

I continue to talk about my perceptions as I see some gray clouds cover up the sky from end to end. I wonder how the sky would look if it was covered with nails instead of clouds. I try very hard to visualize the nails all across the sky, but however hard I try, I get no picture of a nail-covered sky. Some visual pictures are really too difficult to imagine. Yet the picture of a nail-planted wall in that classroom is still so alive that I can describe every detail of it.

And since some pictures are difficult to pull out of memory at the right time and right place, I could not draw a sun when once Mother asked me to draw a sun. I started writing about the sun instead of drawing it. I wrote a paragraph from previously learned information about the sun. Any five-year-old can draw a sun. I could not blame my motor ability for not being able to draw it. I simply could not recall the picture of the sun.

Mother and I worked on the basic skill of drawing diagrams after that. Basic diagrams, like table, chair, sun, clouds, clouds with raindrops, fan, slide, swing, mountains, trees, houses, etc.

Mother said that my learning would be very linear if I

could not produce a basic picture of the object or situation.

So what was the goal of drawing pictures? The goal was to bring my words closer to my real surroundings. I needed to visualize my answers not only in words but also in pictures. And it was necessary to visualize real objects instead of situations of surreal entertainment, like walls filled with nails. I had asked her why.

"Remember how difficult it can be for you to apply your learned knowledge to the components of the environment," she reminded me.

I remembered that I had sat on a sofa many times and Mother would ask me what I wanted to do next. I would answer that I would go get my pencil and write a few lines in my notebook. And I remembered that all those times, I would sit still, without actually getting up and bringing my pencil or my notebook.

My plan to write a few lines remained a mere plan because I could not get the mental map required to actually do anything beyond sitting where I was, or to implement my plan. My pencil and my notebook were in the next room, and I could not map my body to go and bring them, although I could very well visualize the process of opening a page and writing.

Mother asked me to break my plan into step-by-step actions. "First, what do you need to do?" she asked me.

"I need to stand up," I answered.

"So . . . do it," she prompted. Only when she reminded me could I get up.

"Next, what do you need to do?" she asked.

"I need to face the door," I answered.

"Which way is it? Point," she told me when she saw me getting stressed out.

I pointed toward the door. And then I faced the door.

"Now what do you do next?" Mother asked.

"I walk toward the door.'"

"Now do it," Mother prompted again.

I walked to the door from where I could see the next room, where my pencil and notebook were kept. And once I saw them, it became very easy for me to bring them to my writing table.

The purpose of learning how to illustrate my thoughts was to enable me to implement my mental wish by appropriately mapping my activities. In order to do so, I needed to have a basic mental image of the objects and a map representation of my body's orientation in that environment. Things got better with practice. Today, when I tell myself, "I will need the dictionary," I can get a dictionary and not pull any random book off the shelf and get all embarrassed about it.

Once, in a friend's house, I overheard a lady saying that her daughter loved tea. But she wondered whether her daughter knew what a cup and a saucer were because many times she had asked her to fetch a cup and saucer but her daughter could not bring the required things. "Sometimes she would stand in front of the cupboard and look puzzled, and sometimes she would bring the wrong things."

I wonder whether it was because of her mapping problem that she got the incorrect thing.

"But my daughter has no trouble getting the cup when I am pouring tea from the teapot."

"That is because drinking tea is an activity that her voluntary muscles have practiced for many years. So the mapping is done better with that practiced activity. Be sure, lady, that your daughter knows what a cup is."

"Then why can't she bring it when I ask her to bring it?"

"That is because she is not getting or retrieving the right picture of a cup at the right moment. Then, there is her mapping of her actions in the surroundings. She needs to determine which way to turn, which object to reach when there is no tea associated with that object called 'cup,' especially when she can't retrieve the picture."

A Game of Catch

Stories rise and stories break
Stories each and all
Stories formed of memories
Stories big and small.

I could not use a ball in the right way when I was five years old. As a result, although I wished to play with a ball, I was limited in my actions handling the ball. I could just hold it, and if someone asked me to throw the ball, I would jerk my hands and let go of it. The ball would not go very far, although I intended to throw it far toward the person who asked me to throw it. I could kick the ball, too, but it was not quite kicking. I would run toward the ball and one of my feet would touch the ball and push it forward. Yet I loved balls. And I wished to spend time with them. I expressed my wish to Mother by writing it down. I had learned to write before I learned to articulate my words.

One of my speech therapists at All India Institute of Speech and Hearing in Mysore was Mrinal Jha. He devoted part of his sessions to teaching me how to use a ball: throwing, catching, aiming, and all sorts of other ball tricks. While

I practiced handling a ball, a faint wish grew in my mind. It was a faint aspiration, like a gentle breeze around some morning flowers, willing to carry the fragrance a little farther. What if I could handle a ball and got good at it? Would I then be able to play with other children?

I had heard doctors and psychologists ask Mother whether or not I played with other children my age. It made me wonder, too. They said that autistic individuals have trouble playing with other children.

"Perhaps," I thought, "I could play with another boy if I got good at handling a ball." We began at the small therapy park, adjoining the speech therapy clinics on the premises of the All India Institute of Speech and Hearing. Mother and I got a medium-size ball. The ball was the size of an infant's head. When I did not have a therapy session, we worked with the ball. Every time I held it in my hands, it was as if I was holding the head of an infant. I was not to get distracted with the thought of an infant because Mother or Mrinal would throw it toward me, expecting me to catch it, so I needed to be alert.

In the beginning, they would stand very close to me, so that they could drop the ball into my outstretched hands, which were ready to catch it. And I believed that I was actually catching the ball. That belief made me very proud of my ability. And that belief kept me very motivated. I looked forward to the ball-play time with Mother and Mrinal.

I held the ball and beheld it as an infant's head. I felt the pride of perhaps a parent holding an infant. I felt all-powerful with my pride. Sometimes I thought that the sun was also like a ball. It was waiting to drop into my outstretched hands.

I held the ball and did not know what to do with it. I stood with it, not knowing how to throw it back to either Mrinal or to Mother, although I could hear them encouraging me to do so. I would walk toward whoever asked me to throw the ball and place it in his or her hands. I needed to learn how to throw a ball.

One day, Mother got me to stand close to her with the ball, so that we could pass it back and forth between us. Slowly and very gradually, Mother began to distance herself from me, still continuing to pass the ball. To my surprise, I was actually able to throw it back to her from where I stood.

Sometimes I could imagine playing a game of catch with the sun. I would imagine the sun getting tossed from one corner of the sky to another by two pairs of hands. I would wonder about all the shadows getting confused by the restless position of the sun. I would hear myself laugh at the thought of those confused shadows on earth, which wondered where they would fall and how big they would be because the angle of the sun would change so quickly.

"Don't look at the sun so much," Mother would call out

as she held the ball, ready to throw it to me. "You might spoil your eyes."

My hands would get ready to hold the ball or perhaps the sun, as I wondered what those shadows would think if I had to hold the sun in my hands instead of the ball.

I also practiced catch and throw at home. Mother would throw a shirt or a towel or perhaps a potato at me as a substitute for the ball. I needed to stay alert and catch that pretend ball and throw it back at her.

Ball-Man

I saw things through the eyes of a ball. "What if a ball really did have a pair of eyes? And what if it had an opinion of itself? What if it got dizzy because of so much catching and throwing?" I wrote my concerns to Mother.

Mother was motivated by my concerns. She did some serious work on the ball. She drew two eyes and a nose on it. After that, she drew a mouth on that green ball. She also drew two ears on either side. Finally, she scribbled out the hair. "You want a man's head or a woman's head?" she asked.

"Man's," I wrote down.

Mother drew a curled mustache between the nose and the mouth. She was trying to be a perfect artist with the ball. "When we see a rock, we see it just as a rock." Mother continued to chat with me through the ball, pretending to talk to the ball face. "But when an artist sees the same rock, he sees something else, like a winged fairy," Mother continued. "And when I see this ball with my artist's eyes, I behold a face."

Mother continued to be very dramatic with her voice as she held up the ball-face high up in the air as if she was taking a solemn oath. "Thou shalt be a ball-man! And thine eyes shalt witness every rise and every fall as I, thy creator, bounce thy shape up and down, up and down, on the surface of the concrete floor of this room. And wilt thou cry out for mercy and groan of thy pain?"

Mother bounced the ball very dramatically on the floor like Genghis Khan playing with a conquered head. She invited me to join in the bouncing of that mustached ball-man. Then she got more ambitious and fidgety with her pen and the ball. By evening, she had added a beard to that face. And by late evening she added a pair of spectacles to the ball-face. The ball-man uttered no word of protest. I began to feel rather sorry for him. His simple face had too many accessories now.

There was a slide in the therapy park at the All India Institute of Speech and Hearing. I would sit at the top of the slide and watch the ball-man roll down. Sometimes Mother would stand at the bottom of the slide and reroll it upward. Then the ball-man would roll down due to the increasing momentum caused by the slope.

The slide was made of concrete. Its steps and parapet were all concrete. The sliding side was made of polished red concrete. I would throw my green ball-man on it, standing at the bottom of the slide, so that it could bounce back into my hands. As I did this, my reflexes improved every week. I was more prepared for the ball-man to roll down into my hands now.

Mother supervised my ball play, explaining to me the

phenomenon of friction and gravity. Then she explained Newton's laws of motion, as the ball-man rebounded into my hands. I would mentally sing the rock-and-roll song, "Rubber ball is bouncing back to me . . ."

Sometimes, the pen marks on the ball-man's face would fade due to excessive play. Mother would redraw the face: eyes, mustache, beard, spectacles, and all. One day she even stuck two Band-Aids, one on the cheek and one on the forehead, because I would not stop playing with it, even though it was time to go home.

"Ball-man is badly injured." She showed me how injured he was.

"What's Going On Here?"

I needed to learn how to hit a ball with a racket.

My father visited us every four months when we lived in Mysore. He got me a polymer racket and a soft polymer ball, so that I could play at home without damaging the glasses. Hitting a ball with a bat is not something I could wish, then do. It required timing and greater control of my hands, so that I could swing the bat in the direction of the ball.

Mother and I began to practice at home. I include Mother in my learning process, because every time I had to learn a new activity, Mother made me believe that she was learning it, too.

We stood in front of a plywood cupboard, holding the polymer racket in the ready posture. Mother held my hand, which was holding the racket. Mother hit the ball on the cupboard door. The ball bounced back toward us and the racket in our hands hit it back toward the cupboard. We saw the ball bounce back and we hit it again, sometimes toward and sometimes away from the cupboard if we did not hit it right. As the process continued, I began to understand what I was supposed to do.

But before I could take full control of the racket, the landlady who lived downstairs came upstairs. She was holding on to one of her knees. She complained of her arthritis. She came upstairs with her inquiries. She landed upstairs with her frown and questions. "What is going on here?"

The landlady forgot to knock on the door before she entered the room. There was a look of astonished annoyance on her brow. I thought about the brows on the green ball-man's face. His eyebrows resembled a tranquil rolling meadow. The landlady's eyebrows had a more vertical elevation, like two hills. I could picture little mountain goats on them, trying to reach the highest peak. They wished to climb up in the hope of reaching the big red dot, stuck between her brows. Her red dot, the mark of her married status in India, looked like a rising sun on the stretch of her wide forehead, reflecting the summer heat.

I wondered, "Do goats know how to play with a ball?" As I continued to wonder, Mother tried to explain to the landlady why she needed to allow us to practice playing. Mother explained how I had inadequate motor skills and how the ball was very soft and the windows would not break and how she would be very careful to restrict the time to only the evening hours and how once I learned it, she would take the game outdoors because I would then be able to hold the racket and control the ball.

Mother asked her how her arthritis was and whether she would like a cup of tea.

The landlady said that she needed to ask her husband first whether or not we were allowed to play ball inside. And since her husband was out of town that day, we needed to wait till he returned.

Mother needed only to see him entering the gate the following afternoon. "Can we play with this soft ball inside while I am teaching him how to hit it with this bat? I promise not to disturb anyone."

"Sure, you can." The landlord was in a very good mood.

"Only during evening hours!" I heard the landlady's voice complete the sentence.

Mother assured the landlady that she needed to practice other skills too with me, like tying shoelaces and writing. Mother had to cook four meals as well, so beyond evening, she would not find time anyway.

Sometimes Mother would offer the landlady a taste of her curries. The landlady thought them interesting. Otherwise, why hasn't she raised her eyebrows at Mother since then? Why hasn't she raised her eyebrows, even though sometimes the ball-play got wild?

Scattered Senses

As I practiced, I got better with the hand holding the bat. I could even hit a shuttlecock, used in the game of badminton, with my racket. I could hold the bat in my hands for fifteen minutes. Beyond fifteen minutes, the game became more of a chore than entertainment. I could not focus on the shuttlecock for more than fifteen minutes. I would drop the racket and either walk away from it or if I was near my home, I would run inside and stand in front of the mirror. Why would I do that?

I could not tolerate the game for longer than fifteen minutes. My body would feel scattered and my head would be dizzy, which happens even now when I have to be outdoors for long. My body feels more grounded indoors, protected by the four walls of a room. Standing in front of a mirror helps secure my scattered senses.

Sometimes Mother tells me about some of her students, who find it difficult to sit through a long session with continued cooperation. I am sure that they undergo the same overwhelming experience I do when I have to focus all my senses and attention to a task for a long time. I am sure that they, too, experience a scattered feeling of their senses, which makes perceptions, judgment, and planning difficult. It's like a total shutdown of the senses. It is as though the eyes stop seeing and the ears stop listening.

What do I do then? I usually flap my hands to distract my senses to a kinesthetic feel, so that my senses may be recharged. If that worked, I would continue playing badminton for a while. If that failed, I would seek out a more predictable situation where my senses would reconnect in a more meaningful way, so that I could connect my body once again with the environment.

Sometimes, when I am in a social situation, when I have to answer questions while I participate in a dialogue, I might experience a similar feeling — my senses shatter, so it becomes very difficult to continue writing. Writing the next word is like rowing a canoe upstream, when all the pressures and forces are working against you, against my hand holding my pencil.

What would I do then? I would get up in the middle of a sentence, which I began, walk away, recharge my senses with some environmental distraction, and then come back. I would pick up my pencil again and continue with my sentence, thus completing it.

Does this happen to every person with autism? Some may experience it. But I am not sure about everyone experiencing it because most books I have encountered that were written by people with autism were those by high-functioning individuals who can surely function better than me. Or there were books by people who, through facilitation, composed sad poems or poems of love, or have shown anger toward society, making them autism activists. But I am sure some have similar experiences.

The shattered senses can stop all thought processes, making it impossible to continue doing an activity that involves reasoning or using the voluntary muscles of the body.

My playing a game of badminton required a lot of visual focus because I needed to keep a constant eye on the shuttle-cock. That led to a stressed-out visual sense, so even though I wanted to play longer, I could not. It was impossible.

" 'Impossible' is a word written in the dictionary of fools." I remember coming across that famous sentence, once said by some maker of history. He sure was right and he sure was neuro-typical. If someone asked him if it was possible to be on one side of the earth as well as on the other side at the same time, what would he answer?

A similar question was asked by Schrödinger, who invented the wave equation. He asked scientists around the world whether his cat could be alive and dead at the same time if it had to follow the existence of the uncertainty principle of electrons. If Lewis Carroll's Cheshire cat, which would have a smile on its face, was looking at Schrödinger's cat, with the uncertainty of being both alive and dead, it would come to the conclusion that I could be autistic and not autistic at the same time because the uncertainty principle would rule the atoms in my body.

I stand in front of the mirror, looking back at the game of badminton, which Mother and I played on the terrace of the rented apartment, through the eyes of the Cheshire cat. But the mirror has no cat's eye. It shows me another story, a story about jigsaw puzzles.

The Boy Who Does Not Talk but Solves Jigsaw Puzzles

Jigsaw puzzles have become the symbol of autism. Most autism organizations use the logo of the jigsaw puzzle as a metaphor for autism.

Those puzzles occupied a major part of my time during the day and attracted much of my concentration, so much so that I could ignore my shadow if I was playing with them. They could comfort me. They could relax my senses because I was sure what to do with them. I knew which piece to look for and which piece would go where.

I knew that sometimes people watched me. They watched me flap my hands while I looked at my shadow. They watched me walking up and down the street screaming because the street looked strangely indifferent to me. They watched me doing my jigsaw puzzles if they happened to visit my parents for a chat over cups of tea. I never looked at their faces, but I knew that they had their curious eyes on me.

Autism was a new word in India in 1991. It took many years to enter the household teatime discussion of friendly neighbors. People had every right to be inquisitive, and they had every right to be concerned. Why shouldn't they wonder and update their information about me in that small township where my father lived and worked?

After all, nothing much had happened there since Mr. Khan's daughter eloped with a mechanic, who was a poorly waged employee, too junior in status. And they had already gotten bored with gossiping about why the Chatterjees employed a full-time cook. But here before their eyes, I was a phenomenon that was happening, as I was growing big, as I loved to play with shadows instead of with children my age, as my screaming voice got really loud, and as I could also solve jigsaw puzzles.

I knew people watched me work those twenty-piece and thirty-piece puzzles and wonder whether or not I was really smart. Some said that I was smart, while others said that I was smart and spoiled. "Only spoiled children can scream and draw so much attention."

"And if he is really smart, why doesn't he talk?" The next-door neighbor promised to ask her niece who was studying psychology in some college in Punjab. As soon as she knew, she would let my parents know about that budding psychologist's opinion of me.

Once people saw me work with the jigsaw puzzles, they no longer thought that I was mentally retarded. I liked the idea of not being called mentally retarded anymore. I soon became famous in that small township as "the boy who does not talk, but can solve jigsaw puzzles."

I liked the idea of my newly acquired fame so much that whenever guests visited us, I would bring my boxes of puzzles into the middle of the room and start solving them one after another, filling up the entire floor area. I could hear them hushing their conversations and watching me work with a sixty-piece puzzle.

One day, someone had torn up an old page of a typed document and left it on the table to dispose of it sometime in the future. I joined up the pieces, back to a restored page. Things followed after that when someone discovered that I was the one who had restored the pieces of the torn page. It became a source of great entertainment. After that people would give me the torn pages of magazines and watch me join them up into a complete page. I received many more jigsaw puzzles for my next birthday.

However, my first jigsaw puzzle was not so easy for me to solve. My first jigsaw puzzle was inside a blue square box. I still remember Mother opening up the blue square box, made of hard cardboard. It had the logo of the toy company, Fun-school. Inside the box were four puzzles: a four-piece deer, a six-piece lion, an eight-piece elephant, and a ten-piece giraffe.

Mother took out the deer puzzle and broke it up for me, so that I could put the pieces back together and remake it. I looked at the four pieces in a very puzzled way. It hurt to see the deer in four pieces. I wondered whether the mirror upstairs would approve of Mother's actions, so I headed upstairs to see what the mirror thought.

"Where are you off to?" Mother pulled me back toward the puzzle. "Let's see how the pieces get back in place."

I saw the massacred deer in its four pieces. "I am certainly not going to touch it," I decided. I had once touched a piece of a broken porcelain cup and the edges were not smooth. "I am certainly not going to touch those pieces."

I could not talk. Neither could I point out my thoughts on an alphabet chart then. And I could not write because I had not yet learned how to write. So how did I convey my decision to Mother? I pulled myself away from the pieces of the massacred deer.

Mother was now beginning to show her impatience. She placed me on her lap and solved three out of the four pieces. She kept the last piece waiting for me. Because I had already decided that I was not going to touch it, I sat still, not making any attempt to pick up the fourth piece. But my eyes felt the discomfort of seeing that incomplete picture. I expressed my feeling to Mother.

How did I express my discomfort? I pushed Mother's

hands toward the last puzzle piece, hoping she would put it back.

Mother, on her part, pretended not to understand me at all, although I knew that she was faking. She got up and went into the kitchen, as if she suddenly remembered something very important, leaving me alone with that incomplete deer.

I cannot tolerate any kind of distortion. Nor can I tolerate things being out of place. If a chair or a table was out of place, I would immediately place it where it is supposed to be. Guests would find that the moment they rose from their seats, I would immediately reorganize those chairs back in place. And when I was younger, it would distress me to find someone had picked up a magazine from the coffee table because I had arranged them in a certain way. So guests who did not know my habits would be very surprised to find me taking the magazines from their hands and putting them back where I thought they should be. In the kitchen, I would arrange the stainless-steel bowls in neat rows, so that they looked just like those lined-up dates of the calendar.

Mother knew my obsession. Mother knew that I could not tolerate looking at that incomplete picture puzzle for long. I could see her peeping out from the kitchen to see what I was doing with that last piece. That faking woman, pretending to be busy with kitchen work! Why can't she complete it for me? I mentally placed the fourth and last piece of that deer puzzle many times. Yet my hands did not have the courage to touch it.

The puzzle piece lay on the floor, looking up at everything else in that room with patience, hope, and wonder through the eyes of the deer. Mother walked in and out, in and out, trying to keep her feet very busy, while I sat guard, frozen in front of the puzzle. Finally, Mother came in when she saw me get really anxious. How did she know that I was anxious? She saw me flap my hands.

I flapped my hands whenever I got anxious, and Mother did not want me to get anxious. Mother saw me standing in front of the deer puzzle, bending over it as I flapped my hands, to ease away my anxiety through the kinesthetic stimulus, as I wished the deer would stop staring at me.

The deer puzzle lay on the floor, patient, waiting out my anxiety. Mother took my hands. Before I even realized what was going on, she picked up the fourth piece with my fingers, and put it in its place. I saw her hands around my fingers, as my fingers, powered by the pressure of her hands, pinched out the puzzle piece and put it in place.

But before I could sense any relief, she undid the puzzle again. She solved the three pieces, took my hands, and powered my fingers with the pressure of her hold, so that I could pick up the last piece and put it in the right place. As she did this over and over again, I was getting a kind of rhythm to the whole operation. As if in my mind someone was reciting the words,

> "Break them up
> There we go,
> One, two, three, and . . . four,
> Put them back
> Place by place,
> One, two, three, and . . . FOUR!"

My fingers were timed to the word "four."

As I timed my action to the rhythm, it seemed to get more and more easy. My hands began to be sure of the fact that I could pick up the fourth piece at the prompt, "four." I was not scared of the puzzle piece because it did not have sharp edges, as I had thought it would. My eyes memorized every angle of those pieces as my hands, still held by Mother's hand, picked up those four pieces, constructing and deconstructing the deer.

Mother gave my hands more freedom, as they grew less stiff with greater confidence. I recited my mental verse over and over again, as my hands followed the beat.

> "Break them up
> There we go,

One, two, three, and . . . four,
Put them back
Place by place,
One, two, three, and . . . FOUR!"

Did Mother know about the verse I was mentally reciting? No, she did not because I had not yet begun to communicate.

I watched her run upstairs to get her camera, and bring it down to take some pictures of me working with my first jigsaw puzzle. Later I saw those pictures: "my first puzzle piece and I"; the next one was "two solved pieces and I"; the third was "three solved pieces and I"; the fourth was "all pieces solved and I." There were side views of all those stages, and she even took some from behind!

Was I proud? I am not sure. I was finding a new way to stimulate my senses. She was doing all of the fussing. I think Mother was more proud than I that day.

When my father came home from the factory, I had to demonstrate my puzzle-solving ability. Was my father impressed? I am not sure because he did not see the day's drama. Before going to bed, Mother asked me to do another demonstration. I knew she was afraid that I would forget how to do it. Finally, she was at peace when I did it.

Next day, it was the turn of the lion puzzle. The lion had six pieces, and I was no longer afraid of either it or its six pieces. We began the same way, like the deer. Mother solved five pieces, while I solved the last piece. Slowly, we came to the point when the last piece could be any piece. And I was not scared of any piece. In fact, I began to speculate which piece would have its turn as the last piece.

After lunch, Mother solved four out of six pieces, giving me the last two pieces to solve. I felt more and more confident as we proceeded toward solving three, four, and then five pieces, by the time my father came home from work. Before bedtime, I was able to solve both the deer and the lion puzzles.

Was I proud? I am not sure, although Mother kept reminding me that I should be proud of myself. In fact, I was more relieved that I had done them with my very own hands.

Did I get bored of doing just one thing throughout the day? I think not. Because I became more and more ambitious about being able to do it before I went to bed. I think I became obsessive about it. I was sure of what my hands were expected to do, so I felt less scattered with my body. I had a goal in front of me, and I had a vision of that goal. That vision included Mother taking my photographs at the end of the day, which she sure did.

There was no question of getting bored when the ambition was to tame my six-piece lion and be photographed later.

And thus by day
Slow by slow
As time did pass
Years ago,
When hours were spent
With pieces and bits,
I collected them all
To make them fit,
As pictures were broken
As pictures were made.
           I write my moments
           On this page.

Building jigsaw puzzles was a big help to me when this ability was applied to other puzzles, which I loved to solve. How did it help? It helped me through my future IQ tests, when clinical psychologists saw me working on those puzzles.

Mother usually kept me busy during those long waiting times for my psychologist sessions. Usually when I was called, I would be in the middle of a puzzle, and since I would not get up without completing the whole picture, the psychologists would come out into the waiting room to find out what the coaxing was about.

Ever since the psychologists saw me work on the puzzles, they never again said that I was mentally retarded, although they did not hesitate to mention that I had autism. I could tolerate what I have, which is autism. But I could not accept a diagnosis of something that I do not have, mental retardation. I remained thankful to my jigsaw-puzzle-solving ability because I got a better diagnosis, which was honest and acceptable to my ego.

How would a wrong diagnosis affect someone? It would be a blow to his ego and prevent him from being motivated to work hard toward any aspiration. It's like clipping the wings of a bird, which can only look at a treetop but never actually have the means to fly to it.

"Who Knows What I Had Written Down as My Answer to 4 + 2 = ?"

Story, story, one by one,
In from mind, out they come,
In light of day, part by part,
Bit with bit from my past.

I can see myself in a classroom with other members of my class, trying out a simple number problem, wondering why the hell that number 4 has to interact with number 2 through an addition sign.

I go to school because it is too expensive for us to pay for an aide while Mother works during the day. So it really doesn't matter what the special needs program has in store for me during the day. The professionals who work in these programs have their own educational limitations and will have no concept of what coordinate geometry or integration means, let alone how to teach it to any student, regular-ed or special-need. Mother has asked me to tolerate those hours because, after all, it is saving us some money.

As I said before, I was wondering why the hell that 4 had to interact with the number 2, through a + sign. I wondered some more. I looked at the number 2, wondering about the coordinate axes of the plane surface and the probable coordinate points that 2 would hold. And as I saw the position of 2 somewhere on the upper side of the page, I mentally assigned it with the coordinate points of 3 and 7. Three as the x coordinate and 7 as the y coordinate. I could see the page divided into graphic grids.

I heard my aide saying something like I needed to finish up my work. But I was busy assigning a coordinate value to 4. Finally, I settled with the values of 3 and 9 as x and y coordinates. I gave a quick value to the addition sign also. Then I found a whole story of number characters other than merely 2 and 4, competing, quarreling, and asserting themselves to be written down. Finally, I needed the help of "average." I took the average on the x side and the average on the y side to bring peace among the numbers. Who knows what I had written down as my answer to $4 + 2 = ?$

Whatever I had written brought out the very sorry-sounding voice of my aide. "No, Tito . . ." I heard his concerned voice. He was worried about my lack of calculating ability.

I continued to wonder. I was beginning to look at the world of dimensions through the eyes of German mathematician Theodor Kaluza, who worked on his vision about the multidimensional universe. I kept my vision focused on two and four dimensions. What if a two-dimensional point is added to a four-dimensional point? I saw the x and y coordinates of two dimensions overlapping with the x and y coordinates of four dimensions, establishing their components in a strong planar field with a weak z scalar-coordinate axis perpendicular to them. I saw the fourth time-vector coordinate, leading the plane, in a clockwise motion, coming back every twelve hours, in a 360-degree rotation. My day filled with all the exotic wonders that $2 + 4$ could offer. I developed a very powerful $2 + 4$ system, which kept my mind and senses entertained for the rest of the day.

Stories followed more stories around that system when I stood in front of the mirror, which cast back the whole system in an anticlockwise rotation because it had to follow the lateral inversion in order to keep up with its reflecting laws. Sometimes it reflected a $4 + 8$ system and sometimes it reflected a more complicated binary system, which is impossible to explain on the limits of this page.

Learning to Write

Learning to write was the most important skill that I acquired because it helped me to be a storyteller. I had my words and I had my stories, which flowed between me and the mirror. Some stories were absorbed behind the secrets of my shadow, as I watched the shadow through the transparency of my flapping hands.

Some stories lay stretched behind the old buildings and temples of Mysore, as I watched the streets of that old city through my bus window. Stories of a dusty cow and stories of the old bronze statue, stories of the women selling flowers and stories of a monkey sitting on a parapet. I needed to write them down somewhere. I could not possibly use a letter chart to organize all those complicated thoughts. I needed something else to organize my stories.

I needed people to believe that they were my very own stories because I had the proof of my handwriting. If they doubted it, they could see me write my words. I knew very early on in life that if you happen to be born with autism, you will need to give plenty of proofs to doctors, psychologists, teachers, therapists, disbelieving uncles and neighbors, and who knows who else?

Plenty of proof is needed to make those pairs of curious eyes understand that being autistic does not make you a person who just happens to exist, that you are capable of forming opinions about everyone, if they ever found the nerve to hear these. How would they hear if I could not even talk? How would they hear if I was limited to pointing out my words on a letter board, when they were not willing to believe even that?

Many people do not have the patience to see me form words by pointing on the letter chart. Sometimes I pointed to those letters too fast, and sometimes I pointed too slow. The times I went slow, I could feel people were impatient to leave but did not, probably because they did not want to hurt Mother's feelings or perhaps my feelings, if they believed in me at all. Whatever it was, things needed to change. I needed a better way of expression. I did not want to be stuck within the boundaries of a letter board.

Learning a new motor skill like writing meant 80 percent labor, 10 percent motivation, and 10 percent internal resistance. Some days, it meant 50 percent resistance, 50 percent hard work, and no motivation. It was like sailing through a sea that was sometimes calm and sometimes rough.

In the beginning of my first day, I continuously dropped the pencil. I had no problem holding a familiar object in my hands, but due to my selective tactile defenses, holding a new object was a real pain. Every time I held the pencil, I had to focus all of my concentration on the action. My senses were strained by practicing holding the pencil, resulting in discomfort, the kind you feel when the hair of your legs are stroked in the opposite direction of their growth. It was like wearing a new pair of shoes.

Mother had to pick up the pencil every time I dropped it, as I looked at the wall, hoping to get the pencil back. I did it again and again. In fact, I sort of enjoyed the repetition of dropping the pencil and Mother picking it up for me.

Did I want to write? Of course I did.

So why did I drop the pencil again and again, instead of trying to write? When my senses are overstimulated, there is no stopping them. My senses are so heightened that they bury every bit of reason. I was overstimulated by my sensory defenses against the pencil.

How old was I then? I was between five and six years of age, when children my age begin and are settled in their schools. I had just returned from a three-month stay at Christian Medical College Hospital in Vellore. There was no question of my going to any school. Schools in India did not cater to special needs students who did not talk. I had to be at home, educated or not educated.

Mother had made up her mind that we would move to Mysore, away from the interference of disbelieving neighbors and relatives, who had opinions about me but did not have any suggestions for me. In Mysore, there was the All India Institute of Speech and Hearing. And there was Dr. Prathibha Karanth, who was the head of the Department of Speech Pathology. She took a special interest in my well-being, as a person rather than just another case with a speech impairment.

But before we moved to Mysore, Mother wanted me to be able to write. I should be able to write, rather than just point on the alphabet chart, so that I could leave a record of my conversation. We had three months to work toward this goal.

The pages of the notebook fluttered under the air from the ceiling fan. "This is not leading us anywhere," Mother announced as I waited for her to hand me the pencil, so that I could drop it once again. She brought a rubber band from somewhere. She tied the pencil to my fingers in such a way that I could not drop it, even if I shook my hands.

Now that the pencil was secure, I needed to use it. I had to draw lines all across the page. At first, I filled the page with vertical lines. I had always loved to line up matchsticks in rows. Those vertical lines looked like long matchsticks. Mother supervised my movements in the beginning. She did not allow me to free-flow my hands. Vertical lines were meant to be vertical lines and no other shape. Any mistake I made was erased, and I had to draw it again.

Was there any reward? "Rewards are for babies and animals." Mother was religious in her belief.

I got used to the up-and-down movement of my hands as I practiced my vertical lines. Once I was confident with them, I had to draw horizontal lines from left to right. I practiced all morning and all evening. When the pages were full, I practiced on newspapers.

I could feel the pencil as I moved my hands, holding it. Finally, my fingers were no longer tactilely defensive against the pencil. I no longer needed the rubber band.

I began to understand my movements while drawing the lines. Mother made me trace dots on a page, which she drew for me so that my drawing would be more under my control. Sometimes I joined the dots to form zigzags, sometimes triangles, sometimes rectangles, and other times very difficult-to-define shapes. By the end of two or three weeks of day and night tracing I began to love the activity so much that I would wait for Mother to draw more dots on blank pages for me to connect. Soon I found myself joining dots and tracing out alphabet letters. Mother obsessively drew her dotted alphabet letters, while I obsessively joined them.

"We have three months. We have only three months," she kept reminding me. "People need to believe you," she told me every now and then. The idea of urgency was gradually soaking into my mind and pushing my hands to join the dots.

Sometimes we used colored pencils. Other times I used regular graphite pencils. Slowly I began to memorize the motor movements needed to write the letters of the alphabet. Sometimes Mother wrote half a letter, pretending to forget the other half. She would forget to draw all four lines of the letter *M*, or she would forget to draw an arm of the letter *K*. "Something is wrong with this *M* . . . something sure is wrong with the letter *M*," she would mutter as she gave me the pencil for me to join the dots of the incompletely dotted *M*.

By then I had already memorized the motor movements required to write the letter *M*. I would very proudly complete her incompletely drawn letter. Mother would pretend to be very relieved to see the complete letter *M* now balanced on two stick legs, one of which she forgot most probably because she was getting "old and forgetful."

I was filled with pride and vanity because she made more and more "mistakes" on every other letter of the alphabet, and I showed her the mistakes. I enjoyed every bit of it. I realized why people always tell others they are wrong and why they are wrong. I realized that when you correct others' mistakes, it makes you feel superior to them.

Weeks passed. I continued to practice. I progressed as I practiced. I was now copying the letters of the alphabet. I did not need to join the dots anymore. Mother would write words or letters at the top of the page, and I had to copy them. She would write the words *CAR*, *CAT*, and *CAN*.

Sometimes I would do some art by using color pencils or sketch pens. Instead of writing the words, Mother would draw designs on top of the page, using repetitive circles or triangles or curved or straight lines. I had to copy her designs.

Designs always calmed my eyes, perhaps because of their repetitive nature or perhaps because they never questioned my eyes, "Tell me what I am." Drawing or copying a design was very motivating for me.

As I practiced my pencil control, my confidence grew. In three months I was sure of my handling the pencil. I was good at tracing and copying. Mother reintroduced the letter board to me once I had mastered copying.

"Spell out the word *CAT* for me on this board."

I touched the letter *C*.

"Now copy *C* on your page." Mother gave me the paper and pencil.

I copied *C*.

"What comes next?" Mother asked me.

I touched the letter *A*. She handed me the pencil again to copy *A*, next to *C*.

"What comes after *C* and *A*?" Mother showed me the letter board.

I touched *T*. She handed me the pencil and I copied *T*

after *C* and *A*. I looked at my first word and felt extremely confident in my hands.

More words followed in the same way, and many more words followed in the days after.

This was a new way to use the pencil. I became more and more confident. I knew that I would be believed because I could write on my own, and Mother would not need to be my scribe anymore. I spelled and copied more words on the page in front of me. Every page shone with my relief and confidence. Every word that formed in my mind was written down by my own ambitious hands on the pages of the notebooks where I practiced every day.

As a rule, Mother saw to it that I wrote every day, in the morning, before I did anything else. I continue to follow this rule today without missing a single day.

Writing became a natural discipline in my life. Slowly, I got used to writing down the letters from memory instead of copying them letter by letter. I would spell the words first, then Mother would cover up the letter board so that I could write that word from memory. If I got stuck, she would show me the letter board again and ask me to touch the letters once more and write them down. There was no longer any pressure on me.

Letters were written
Words were formed
Step by step
I moved on
With my words
Short or long.

Divine Phenomenon!

Equipped with my words and my writing skills, I came to Mysore, where I would be meeting more psychologists who would do many more tests on me. I looked forward to showing them what I could do.

Mother rented a small one-room apartment, where we ate, worked, slept, and cooked. I continued to practice my writing, which steadily progressed with my increasing confidence. I could write my own stories and poems. There was no question of people believing me because they saw my words in my handwriting and not in my mother's handwriting.

I turned six. Some people in Mysore thought I was a divine phenomenon. "Otherwise, why should he be able to write and not speak?" they argued with Mother when she tried to tell some of her new friends that I had autism. In India, the word *autism* is relatively new.

"Whatever -isms you may call it, you must believe that no one can write without speech."

I began to wonder myself whether I really was some kind of divine phenomenon. At home Mother told me, "Divine phenomenon or any other phenomenon . . . you need to work hard so that your writing develops."

I began to miss the upstairs mirror, which I had left back home. I believed that it could show me what I was. In this new home we had a smaller mirror, and I had yet to befriend it.

Every day I would go for my speech therapy sessions at the All India Institute of Speech and Hearing. We would come back from the institute and work on writing for fifteen minutes at a stretch, followed by a ten-minute break. I would come back to our work mat and write for another fifteen minutes, then take another break. This continued till dinner. In the first few months of my writing, I could not write for more than fifteen minutes at a time. My eyes got dazed and the hand holding the pencil felt heavy as a rock.

I could write more in the mornings, before leaving for the institute. I would complete an article about a cow I saw the previous evening, or a poem about an anthill, or a story about the unplastered wall of bricks on which I saw a monkey sitting and looking at the sun, although I believed that it was actually looking at me and only pretending to look elsewhere. I would not get up without completing my article. And I never looked at the time, or how long I wrote, in the mornings.

I got my first offer to be published at the age of six and a half in a quarterly magazine called *Beehive*, which was run by a group that worked for nature conservation awareness. They selected four of my poems, although I wished they had selected all. The poems were of six- to eight-line rhyming stanzas that I wrote about forests and birds.

"How can they select all?" Mother asked me. "Don't they have other articles to put in their pages?"

It was a beautiful, glossy, blue-covered magazine. In other words, it was very impressive. There were pictures on most pages. On the cover, there was a photograph of the white Himalayas against the blue sky — a part of the earth reaching up to touch the sky. The cover became my source of inspiration, then it turned into an obsession. I would mentally sit on the mountaintop and look up at the sky. I could feel the triumph of achievement. For my words were printed. I needed to write more, and I needed to write better.

By now I was friendly with the new mirror in my Mysore home. I would see the magazine reflected in it. "If you dangle that magazine, can you imagine what will happen to it?" Mother was very concerned about my holding the magazine by the corner of the cover page.

I heard her and I heard her not.

I was hearing the silence of the mirror, which was reflecting Mother's words, "If you wish anything with both your heart and mind, Nature will use all her powers to help you!"

"Now why should anyone sniff those pages?'" Mother was letting me know that pages are not for sniffing.

I heard her yet I heard her not.

Writing Down Dictated Words

At the All India Institute of Speech and Hearing, my speech therapist, Mrinal Jha, found out that I had trouble taking dictation, although I had no problem writing words I thought about on my own. I could write the word *house* when it originated in my mind, but I just could not picture that word when he asked me to write it. When given the letter board back, though, I could spell it very well because the letters were right in front of my eyes and I needed no extra effort to bring them forth from memory.

Some people who saw their children pointing and spelling may wonder, "Why should anyone be worried about this problem?" Wasn't pointing and spelling on the letter board or a keyboard enough?

I was worried about my problem. Why couldn't I get the picture of the word *house* when Mrinal asked me to write it down? I was lucky to have such an observant speech therapist. Not only was he observant, he was also ambitious about my progress. And I am glad that Mother and he worked together toward my new goal, writing words, then writing down dictated sentences.

There are certain things that can puzzle people who are

dealing with autism. My state still puzzles me. Why would it not puzzle others?

One learned skill does not lead to another skill even if it is similar to the learned skill. For example, knowing the spelling of a word and being able to recall it immediately when necessary may not go hand in hand. It may require the help of a familiar condition. By which I mean, how the word or phrase was learned and what the environmental conditions were when the learning took place.

Is learning a skill complete if it cannot be applied to other conditions? It is necessary to be able to apply a skill. No one wants to be embarrassed when people do not believe in one's ability to perform a skill because of an inability to apply it to other situations.

Many times, I am sure neuro-typical people ask whether any understanding is going on in the minds of people with autism. That is because the learning of the required skill is not demonstrated in the way a typical person expects.

I get very embarrassed when I cannot perform a task, even though I've performed a related task.

Here, the related task was pointing and spelling a dictated word on a letter board, but I could not write down the dictated word from memory, even though I could use this word in my poems or other texts, when not dictated.

Wondering about my problem, or worrying about it,

would not help anyone in any way. I needed to do something about it. I needed to learn dictation as a completely new skill. With every new skill I learn, more areas of my brain are exercised. New pathways are established by new activities. Learning a new skill begins with crawling steps and a combination of motivation and resistance.

Mother would come home and draw diagrams to show me what my nerves were doing when I struggled with taking down dictated words. On the first few days, she would draw the dendrites and make a chain of them. She would draw them very lightly to show a feeble connection among them. As days passed, she would show a darker connection between them because they were supposed to be gaining in strength as I practiced. I could imagine the neurons making a pathway in my brain, as I showed more motivation and less resistance.

Mrinal worked on my dictation-taking skill. He began by dictating words with the same suffixes. For example, all words ending in -at, like *cat, bat, fat, mat,* and so on, so I could concentrate only on the first letter of that word. By the end of the session, I would be able to write all those words, dictated in any order, without referring to the letter board. How long was my session? It lasted for one hour.

Mrinal passed on the list of ten words to Mother, so that she could have me practice them at home. To be honest, it was boring to practice the same words over and over again. But Mother assured me that it was necessary because who knows at which point of my life I would be asked to demonstrate it.

Once I mastered those words, we moved on to words ending in -an, like *pan, ran, can, fan,* and so forth. I not only needed to write them down without the assistance of the letter board, but I had to write them down with Mrinal or Mother sitting in another part of the room, at least two feet away from me.

From three-letter words, I moved on to bigger words. For example, four-letter words ending in -ond, like *bond, pond, fond,* etc., which later helped me extend to words like *beyond* and *second.* From same-suffixed word dictation, I began taking down words beginning with the same prefixes, like *brand, branch,* etc. Later, I practiced conjunctions, like *although, because, since,* and so on. I could almost see the neurons in my brain, collectively helping me write those dictated words and sentences. I no longer felt insecure without the letter board, or Mother or Mrinal sitting close to me.

With repetition and practice, I could write many words with fluency when dictated or when not dictated. I was no longer a slave to the letter board. Since I could write now, it was easier to answer the different tests that awaited me in different places and countries in the years to come.

I first tasted writing's fruits when I turned eleven years

old and was invited by the BBC and the National Autistic Society in the United Kingdom, halfway across the world, and was tested by Lorna Wing, Judith Gould, and Beate Hermalin. And since I could write my answers and thoughts, I was believed.

I was believed by those legends of autism research. Who cared whether or not those new psychologists and psychiatrists back in India believed me! And who cared why some skeptic aunt or cousin found me weird! And since those researchers believed me, my first book, *Beyond the Silence* (released in the United States as The *Mind Tree*), was published. Not only was I published, I was also told that the BBC documentary on me, *Tito's Story*, won the Emma Award in Britain.

I can thank my luck for having such great speech and language therapists at the All India Institute of Speech and Hearing in Mysore, who looked beyond their fields of articulation and speech production to give their time toward my longtime goal, which was not just speech production but to be believed.

It Worked Better than a School

Going to the All India Institute of Speech and Hearing worked better for me than going to any special school. Dr. Prathibha Karanth was my mentor and counselor, while speech therapists worked on my specific goals.

I never have to worry about education, for Mother always educated me, at home as she still does. But after coming to the United States and after Mother got a fellowship, then a job offer, I attended a school designed for special needs students in Los Angeles. The special school focused on social modification of behavior and social adaptation in various circumstances through behavior training. There was no educational expectation, because it was believed that education is the right of individuals who can voice their language.

Am I criticizing a belief adopted by different schools? No, I am not. But how will people know how to teach someone who has language and yet manifests his thoughts in such alternate ways that are classified as bad behavior?

Why couldn't I and others like me display good behavior? The answer is this. Behavior is a social activity. Social activities arise from the hypothalamus of the brain. From there, the impulse travels to the body, where there is a change in heart rate or a flow of adrenaline or some other hormonal activity. The impulse is then sent back to the brain, where it passes to the premotor cortex, then the motor cortex — a very long pathway. Due to the underconnectivity of my neurons or some alternate connectivity, instead of performing the socially required task, like smiling at a familiar person, I may perform an alternate task, like picking up a book and sniffing.

Struggling Our Way Out of a Belief System

My most difficult years were in Los Angeles when I was standing on the threshold of puberty, between the years 2001 and 2004.

There was a nagging thought on my mind. There was this continuous reminder that something was wrong somewhere. I felt that Mother and I were thinking in two different directions. Mother was involved in the activities of organizations that were raising money for researchers to find a cure for autism. I had no problem with the research part. Certainly, research was necessary to understand the mind of an autistic person. I wondered about the promises of a cure.

I was astonished by Mother's involvement with the belief that autism is a disease and needs a cure. Mother had always believed in my thoughts and judgment before. How could she participate in a system that classified me as sick? Did Mother really think I was less of a person?

We had a talk. Mother and I had to find a way out of the sickening web of this belief system. After two years in this system, we felt suffocated because it policed our every move, prevented opportunities for interviews, and signed away the rights to our story on our behalf, without even having the courtesy of consulting us. Something is wrong somewhere. There was a series of wrong judgments, wrong feelings, and wrong events. Everything looked wrong everywhere. We were at the bottom of a well surrounded by the high wall of the belief system that we could not be part of. Watching the waters of the ocean from the shore is different from being in it day after day, knowing that we are creatures of the land and do not belong here.

I do not criticize any person or his efforts toward the belief system. I simply was not a part of it because I believe in the dignity of my belief.

Mother and I served that system of belief as long as our contract lasted. In fact, we served it a year and half more, out of gratitude and goodwill, till we felt suffocated by its demands.

Everything looked wrong everywhere.
The sky looked blue
The buildings of Hollywood
Got shaped by the daylight
Or artificial neon lights by night
Red, green, or blue,
Yet everything looked wrong everywhere.

Mother and I had to find our own path somewhere. That somewhere had to be a place away from Los Angeles.

"I Need You to Prescribe Me
Some Medicine"

My story remains in a state of idle wonder, as I sit in our Austin home, thinking about every experience that mattered in my life. I include every milligram of Risperidal which my psychiatrist, Dr. Dickstein, prescribed to me during those troubled days in Los Angeles.

Dr. Dickstein was a doctor for the county. He had read every page of my published book, and continued to read my other writings as well. He prescribed me necessary doses of Risperidal. This drug helped me to pull my mind out of the trap of my paranoid state, for I became suspicious of everyone around me, including those who cared most about me, like Arnel and Mother.

I stopped answering e-mails because I wanted to have nothing to do with computers. I was suspicious of the shadows around me at night, finding it difficult to close my eyes and sleep. To my utter disappointment, stories would not form around any of those breathless shadows, as I could feel them mauling my body, trying to squeeze sleep from my eyes with the hissing whisper of "everything is wrong everywhere." I could not shut my eyes and go to sleep.

Shadows stretched beyond through the quiet
In the dreamless wake of the hissing night.
They stared at each sigh and each breath
Like the open eyes of the swallowing gates of death.

"Mother, I need to go for a walk." I woke Mother. I had to wake her.

"But it is only two A.M.," Mother said in a sleepy voice. "Can we go in the morning?"

"I cannot wait, I just cannot wait," I heard my voice saying, and I heard the walls echo back from all four directions, knocking the front door with louder voices, resounding back, "I CANNOT WAIT, I JUST CANNOT WAIT."

I saw my flapping hands trying to shake away the hold of the clasping night around my wrists and fingers. I felt a choking sensation around my throat, as my voice grew loud and impatient, threatening a scream. I picked up the keys as Mother finally got up.

There was no choice for Mother. She had to open the door. There was no choice for me either. I was scared of my own self that felt all choked up in the denseness of the sleepless night, and I felt the need to scream out my suffocation at any moment.

"We are just going around the block, and then you are going straight back to bed," Mother warned me. "All these

strange ideas come to your mind. . . . Tomorrow I have to
work all day. . . . How am I supposed to work when I don't
get sleep? Tomorrow I am calling Dr. Dickstein," Mother
muttered and grumbled along. "I can't allow all these fancy
ideas to come again."

> I heard her and heard her not.
> I was breathing in the life
> Around Hollywood Boulevard
> For many eyes around me
> Were open, as people walked,
> And laughed or talked.

> I looked around me
> At those open restaurants
> And at the streets,
> At the waking lampposts and
> At those tall palm trees
> At the empty sky above my head
> While Mother and I
> Walked step after step.

> I began to enjoy every fragment of the night.
> For Hollywood Boulevard was awake like we were

It felt like 7 P.M.
Even when the clock showed a little after 2 A.M.
People walked out of the cinemas and restaurants.

There were people standing
Under the mysterious shade of closed shops,
There were girls giggling at each other
Or who knows what?
One of them came near me and
Asked me the time,
Although I did not wear my watch.

"He is my son, and he is autistic."
Mother tried to push me ahead
Because my footsteps had stopped.
"What is your problem?" the girl asked her back.

We heard her
We heard her not.
Mother wanted to turn back home
I wanted to walk.
Mother followed my footsteps
Lest I get lost,
I wanted to escape the night
At all cost.

"We should do this walk every day," I suggested to Mother.

Perhaps Mother had looked at me in surprise, or perhaps she had looked at me with annoyance. I did not see her eyes as we came inside our apartment. And she did not answer.

I did not or could not sleep for three nights in a row. For all those nights, like a holy pilgrim, I kept my steps going back to Hollywood Boulevard at 2 A.M. One day I wondered where that solitary violin player lived. The next day I looked around for those giggling girls, one of whom had asked me the time. Will I ever recognize her? I never saw her again.

After three days, we got an appointment with Dr. Dickstein. Dr. Dickstein wanted to know why I could not sleep.

From my previous experiences with psychology-oriented people, I have learned not to pour out my heart when they ask something. I have learned through my experiences with other psychologists and psychotherapies that psychologists have a strange belief that they can change the circuits of the brain and perhaps the chemical processes in the brain by listening to the client, with their wisdom and confidence. And I have also learned that they will not leave you alone until they get you to confess that your belief or action is not correct if it doesn't match their belief system. So when Dr. Dickstein asked me why I could not sleep, I wrote down that I wondered about that, too. And I wondered what medications he would prescribe.

What was the use of telling him? Very few people understand my partial synesthesia when I cannot think and analyze the different aspects of my environment in a rational manner, so there was no use explaining to anyone how the dimensions of the night can enter one's mind and become so alive that it can squeeze out the last drop of sleep from one's eyes, leaving it thirsty like a desert.

"I just need you to prescribe me some medicine," I wrote.

I loved the look on the doctor's face. He looked at me with more respect and trust than I ever saw in any medical professional's eyes. But I had to answer his questions first because there was no single medication for sleeplessness.

After he saw my answers, he told me that I was experiencing a state of acute hypomania, where I suffered from extreme obsession and an overalert mind. That was why I was suspicious of shadows and people.

The very thought of my mind makes me wonder at its mysteries. What else is a mind but a mysterious possession, which allows all those fortunate and unfortunate things to be experienced, giving us the gift of either pleasure or pain? And what is a mind which is controlled by an obsession, causing all other thoughts to be shrouded under its pressure and cover?

Obsessions to Count

My obsessions were many.

How old was I then? Perhaps seven or eight.

I was obsessed with looking up at the blazing sun in India, even though Mother tried to distract my view toward other things. I would look at the sun until my eyes were so dazzled that when I turned them toward something else, they still held the impression of the sun. And that impression stayed for a while. Then, as it grew fainter and fainter, I would go outside and look at the sun again.

When I turned nine I was obsessed with adjusting my belt and my shirt collars. Mother overlooked this because it did not matter much to onlookers on the streets and bus stops.

I was obsessed by the swing, which, in my mind, stood waiting for me to sit on it whenever I went to the Spastic Society of Karnataka in Bangalore. I was eight when we moved there, and they allowed me to use their campus during the day. I was invited to sit in the classes, but most of the time, I chose to sit on that swing. I would rock on the swing, and let it rock me, to and fro. I would hear Mother giving me a science lesson on simple pendulums and the harmonic motions. Yet I would rock, to and fro. I would put words to every to and fro movement until they resounded in my ears like a poem. I would go home and write down those words. Mother did not stop me from that obsession either, for she was eager to see me write.

When I came to Hollywood, I got some new obsessions. One was riding a metro bus to a certain destination, and then returning by the metro underground train to the Hollywood Highland station. From there, I would walk back home. It became my daily ritual.

How strong was this obsession? I felt like I was inside a plastic box, suffocated all day long, until I could take those metro bus rides. I could not imagine myself not riding the metro bus and train, even for a day.

When did I take those rides? After school. Every day, after Arnel accompanied me back home, I urged him to take me to the bus stop. And what if he did not? I am sorry to say, that I would have a temper tantrum, which was beyond my control.

Why was I obsessed and why did my obsession affect my behavior? I cannot explain it from a psychological point of view, but I can certainly explain it through neuroscience.

An obsession begins in the caudate nucleus in the brain. From the caudate nucleus, the impulse passes to the pre-frontal cortex. From the prefrontal cortex, the impulse goes to the cingulate cortex. The impulse from the cingulate cortex goes back to the caudate nucleus, thus completing a cycle. The cycle repeats again and again inside the mind. So an obsessive impulse is not easy to distract.

Why does it bring an extreme manifestation of behavior? That is because the caudate nucleus is so close to the amygdala region of the brain, which is responsible for all our primitive emotions, like fear and anger. When the caudate nucleus is stimulated, the amygdala is also affected.

My extreme obsession with train rides was beyond my reason and control, although I understood that I was being irrational about it. It is the same process that goes on in the mind of perhaps a chain-smoker, who, although he knows and understands completely well that he is not supposed to smoke, is still compelled to.

During the day, while still in school, I mentally took many trips on the metro bus and the metro train. I had to spend several hours in that special school in Los Angeles, with a pair of scissors and colored paper because I was supposed to make some decorative cards for one of those holidays when you are supposed to give cards to one another. I was never a good planner or maker of cards, and I knew that my aide Arnel would help me to complete it. So why bother? Why not keep my mind occupied with some better entertainment?

How did I entertain my mind? I took several trips on the

metro bus and the metro train. I was interrupted many times as I mentally tried to remember every cross street, every store, and every tree that passed my way if I sat by the window of the bus. And each time I was interrupted, I had to start all over again because I would lose track of where my bus ride had stopped. It made me upset, and if it happened with greater frequency, it caused a few outbursts. I knew very well that the mental bus ride was not a realistic goal. But what else could I think of when my hands were holding crayons or glue or a pair of scissors, making cards for who knows what event? I was not visual enough to have any idea how my card should look. I don't believe in getting or giving cards because of my old-fashioned mind, which believes more in genuine letter-writing. Cards look too superficial and formal to me.

As I took my mental bus and train trips, my mind began to race further beyond my control. Sometimes it surprised me. Sometimes it sucked all my thoughts and reason, bringing them inward with giant velocity. I was scared of it. I had to stop my obsession.

My writing did not please my ears anymore. It was not that I did not write, even while I tried to fight the obsessive thoughts of those rides. But writing became a mere duty or a task, rather than an ambition to please my ears and satisfy my heart. I wrote pages of rubbish. I was embarrassed by my own work. Incomplete prose and poetry sounded hollow in my ears after Mother read them aloud. Completed poetry was of inferior quality. Those incomplete stories waited to be told and finished.

I stood in front of the mirror, but I could see nothing beyond my physical reflection. Colors and stories no longer formed behind it. I tried to complete my stories by standing in front of it, but the all-consuming thought of the train and bus rides sucked my imagination with its strength, vacuuming my mind clean. My frustration knew no bounds.

I have seen certain plants thriving in a certain type of earth. They do not thrive in other types of soil, however much energy one may put into maintaining them by providing the proper humidity and temperature the plant needs.

I was like one of those plants.
I belonged to a different garden.
There was nothing wrong with the city of Los Angeles.
But it was not for me.
It had everything in it.
It had a great volume of energy and stimulation.
It had the sounds,
It had the lights,
It had its stars
And all its wonders.
Many had found their dreams in it.

For it had everything in it.
There was nothing wrong with the city of Los Angeles,
But it was not for me.
I was one of those plants,
I belonged to a different garden.

Risperidal helped me for a while by at least allowing me to
sleep through the nights and be less suspicious of people. But
I realized that I needed a different environment. I needed a
quieter and slower environment. I was more than relieved
when I heard Mother discuss moving to Texas, to the city of
Austin.

So those stories, here or there,
Stretch away through air or earth,
Some of this, mixed with that,
Like flowers or thorns in my gypsy heart.
They bloom and prick, now and then
In my heart, from their stem,
As I write them down with words,
Those stories of my gypsy heart.

Power Outage in the Metro Rail

I miss many faces from Los Angeles. I remember my aide Arnel's face. Arnel was my aide between the years 2001 and 2004. I see his understanding eyes, coping with my worst temper tantrum that day the metro train stopped due to a power breakdown.

The train was heading downtown. It was crowded, and the compartment looked like a container filled with faces and bodies, sitting or standing, anxious to go home after work. Everything looked normal, and everything corresponded to my mental map.

What is a mental map? A mental map is a mental picture I form, which I expect to face in the process of events, so that I am not surprised or shocked by any sudden situation. Sudden situations, which invade my mental map, are like meteors hitting a sublime corner of a peaceful planet. And just like the meteor's impact on the planet, the suddenness of an unknown situation creates an unpleasant effect on my mind. It creates anxiety and, like a chain reaction of nuclear fission, it continues to blast all around my mind, so that instead of a peaceful thought process taking place, all that happens is the combined destruction of one blast after another.

Suddenly, the train stopped and the lights went out. There was a small emergency light, but that little lamp increased the density of the crowd, closing up the spaces between people with intense and mysterious shadows. Shadows crept around, climbing on the faces of people. And shadows crept around my feet, as they climbed around my body with slimy determination. I could feel those shadows on my breath, forcing me to breathe in their sliminess. I felt suffocated under their forced pressure. I felt the need to breathe in air. And I felt the need to go outside.

Going outside was not easy because all the doors were locked. Looking out through the windows was not helpful at all inside that dark tunnel, where the metro train was standing like a dead soul, inside the pathway to hell, waiting for its turn to go in.

What did I do in that state of extreme panic and claustrophobia? I remember turning around and looking from side to side. I remember seeing the opaque shadows and opaque faces to my left and right. I remember hearing an infant crying somewhere close by or perhaps far away. And I remember the sound getting entangled in the heavy breaths in that patch of darkness. I remember no movement, other than my head in patches of dark. I felt my aching lungs, and then feared that my heart might stop. I felt the touch of Arnel's strong hands, holding on to my shoulders, as I tried to break the wall of people and faces with my hands, my head, my knees, so that I could reach the shut door of that compartment. I felt Arnel's hold all around my body, protecting my limbs, lest they act unfaithful to my soul. His hold remained till the power in the train was restored and the train started moving.

"How long was the power gone in the train?" Mother asked Arnel when we got home.

"Fifteen minutes," he answered.

My view of the metro train ride changed after that. One patch of black ink can spoil the look of a page filled with neatly written words. And that one experience was enough to stop my urge to go for train rides every day.

Every time I sat in the classroom of that special school in Los Angeles and thought about the train ride, I could only relive the experience of acute claustrophobia. I would get up from my seat and try to walk out of that room in the basement, which was my classroom. What would happen after that? Arnel would try to stop me, and I would feel suffocated once again because the classroom would turn into a train compartment with slimy shadows around people and their faces.

You might wonder exactly what I did to display my anxiety. I wonder myself. All I can say is that I recall the urge to hold on to anything within arm's reach. My body starts feeling numb, and my throat feels extremely dry. My diaphragm is pushed up and squeezes the breath out of my lungs. I feel like my breaths are not enough to complete the respiration process, and I take shorter and faster breaths, so that my lungs can continue to pump in oxygen. That is what I experience.

Reaching the Other End

Happenings. They happen all the time. What else is time, if it does not cover happenings? Some of these happenings are noticed, while others go unnoticed. And what gets noticed depends on the intensity of that happening.

Once, I was visiting this really big house in Los Angeles. I was in one of its rooms, which had a high ceiling, many doors, and several pictures on the walls. Every space in that room was filled with something. There were many people around me, some of whom, I was told, worked in the movie industry.

Why was I there? I was a close friend of the lady of the house, who was involved with autism and believed in devoting her energy to finding a cure. Although I had a different opinion, I still considered her a friend. Because I was a friend, I was there with Mother.

My knowledge about movies was inadequate to appreciate the movie workers. I grew up exposed to the works of Keats, Shelley, Byron, Hardy, and Dickens, so the presence of workers in the entertainment industry did not arrest my attention. The intensity of the energy in that room was very strong. I felt like a small raft floating in the midst of the energy in that room. The energy bounced across the room, all around the walls, the pictures reflected them, and the tables diverted them toward the ceiling. Every corner demanded my attention, as I could actually see the pathway of the energy wave, bouncing around with speed. Voices competed with voices. The colors of the clothes and dresses worn by people competed with each other. Even the pictures on the walls seemed to compete with each other for my attention. What do I hear and where do I look?

My dominant sensory channel is hearing. It dominates to such an extent that I dream in sounds most of the time, even when I sleep at night. So if anyone asks me, "What did you see in your dream?" I would answer, "I heard my dream."

I tried to listen to their talk, to distract my eyes, which were bouncing from corner to corner, following the energy pathway, and were now getting tired. I could hear nothing but social talk from voices, which slowly formed a collective tunnel around me. I could gradually see the tunnel turning solid around me, as more voices gathered to shape it. Its opaqueness prevented me from seeing the wall or the ceiling or the bouncing energy across the room that I had seen before. I saw myself in that tunnel, within its diameter. I could see one of the doors of the house at the other end of the tunnel. The door was predictable, and it promised freedom.

Feeling claustrophobic, I began to walk toward the door,

where the tunnel ended. As I walked to the door, I could perceive the tunnel around me being piled up with more and more sounds of greetings and laughter. I had to escape that trap.

"Why did you cross the street and go to the house in front?" Mother asked me.

I realized that Mother had followed me. I was surprised. It seemed to me as though I was crossing the tunnel so that I could see the light and breathe in fresh air. Little did I know or realize that the door I was seeing on the other end of that tunnel was the door of the house across the street. Little did I realize that I had crossed the street to come to that door.

I heard Mother's voice next to my ear sounding puzzled at my leaving the room and ignoring the fact that there was a street. The very sound of her voice melted the tunnel back into the transparency of the physical world, abiding by the rules of Nature.

I have heard of people walking in their sleep and doing many things without having any recollection of what they did. I cannot compare my experience to sleepwalking. That is because I was very aware of what I was experiencing while I believed I was crossing a tunnel.

I had to do my own research on why it happened that way. I had to do my own research because if I told anyone, they would say that I was imagining it. Yet the experience was so real that I can replay it any time. After reading certain texts on neuroscience, I have come up with a suitable answer.

Experiences are stored in the mind, broken into components. These components are language units, belief units, emotion units, action units. These units must interact with each other to recall the experience in the right way. By the right way, I mean, parallel to the happenings.

Happenings in the same environment can be many, involving one or several components in that environment interacting with one another. For example, the light from a lamp above and the air from a table fan, falling and interacting with this page on which I am writing. While I am writing, many other happenings are also taking place around me, like the moving needles of the wall clock, which perhaps my senses are not noticing because my senses are not interacting with them at the moment. I am aware of the light falling on this page, which I feel is too harsh. I come to that conclusion only after I compare it with past experiences of other lights falling on pages, which my memory recalls.

As my mind goes beyond the physical definition of light and air, I can easily transfer my thoughts to some other observation, far from physical interpretation. So it is very natural for me to feel that the air from the table fan is trying to blow away some of the intensity of the light from the surface of this page. Although it is not physically happening, it is the story my mind has formed. While I experience this situation, I am also putting my thoughts into language, so I can write them down exactly as I experience it. As I am writing it down, I am wondering how I will recall this situation, if necessary, ten years from now, since this experience will be stored in my memory, which is broken into four components: units of language, units of belief, units of emotion, and units of action. The same experience may be stored and interpreted by another person in a different way, depending on how his units of memory were stimulated.

"Tell Us What He Was Reading"

I was in a research laboratory in San Francisco. "Tell me what I was reading about," Claude asked me in one of those rooms, which had stacks of files, old desktop computers on every table pushed against the walls in all directions, and large office chairs around a large center table. Those chairs were occupied by people whose eyes were turned toward me.

Who knows what he was reading about? I was aware that I was supposed to hear what he was reading. I was aware that I would be asked questions from the passage he was reading. And I was also aware that I did hear him. The difference is that I heard his voice more than I heard his words.

Claude read. I heard his voice fill up the spaces between the files and dig behind the computer monitors. I saw the voice transform into long apple green and yellow strings, searching under the tables for who knows what? Threads like raw silk forming from Claude's voice.

Claude read. I watched those strings vibrate with different amplitudes as Claude tried to impress the silent beholders and serious researchers of autism with the varying tones of a near-to-perfection performance.

Claude read. I watched those strings with stresses and

strains, reaching their own elastic limits and snapping every now and then, when his voice reached a certain pitch. I saw those snapped strings form knots like entangled silk, the color of apple green and yellow.

Claude read. I heard his voice, and saw its vibration blowing away those silk threads all over the floor.

"So what was he reading?" a voice asked me again when Claude closed his book. I saw all those strings, snapping all at once around his mouth, making a remarkable effect around his face in yellow and green. Someone handed me a piece of paper and a pencil, so that I could write. Although I did not attend to what Claude read, I did write about the beauty of the color green, when yellow sunshine melts its way through newly grown leaves.

Why did I write that, instead of just writing that I had not listened to his passage? I wanted to be honest in my own way about my experience of that situation, as my perception was interpreting it to me when translated into language. Those apple green and yellow strings produced by his voice reminded me of fresh leaves and yellow melting sunshine like fresh butter.

Mother knows my difficulty of overassociation when she reads. So when Mother reads to me, she pauses every now and then, after one or two sentences or three sentences, depending on the length of those sentences and the amount of information each has to impart, and asks me to explain what I understood.

I need to be alert because she will not proceed if I do not answer her, and I will have to hear the same sound in words again and again. I have no choice but to pay more attention to her words because my experience of listening must be more toward the content of the passage and not the effect produced by her voice. Otherwise, instead of listening to what I am supposed to hear, I might experience what I did when Claude was reading.

I find myself or someone else with autism reacting to a situation in an alternate way, which may be different from the socially expected norm. It may be unique to me or to the other person with autism, depending on which component unit is more dominant in a given situation. When I pick up a book, I might turn the pages and sniff each page first before looking at the pictures in it because I believe in finding out first, as a ritual, how old that book is and how many hands have turned the pages of that book before me. Someone else with autism may tear a page or two, for who knows which dominant unit of experience is taking place in his perception. Another person with autism may totally ignore the presence of that book because his perceptions would be directed toward some other aspect of the environment, and his experience would revolve around that component. Each brings forth a unique manifestation of overt action, which psychology defines as behavior.

I have seen many people with autism write about themselves, claiming that they can understand every aspect of the dynamic environment in its every detail and blaming only their motor dysfunction for not being able to perform. Maybe they do. I don't.

I do not believe that only my motor dysfunction is to be blamed for my alternate actions, which others call behavior. I tend to overinclude many components within or outside the limits of my surroundings into the permeability of my mind, often resulting in a tangential way of perception.

Do I voluntarily involve extra components to existing components in the environment, like those green and yellow strings around Claude's voice? No, I don't. Those extra components are totally beyond my voluntary control. On that particular day my overassociative mind allowed me to perceive Claude's voice in strings of green and yellow. Why, I wonder, were they green and yellow and not just green, or pink and blue? I do not know.

Do I perceive strings whenever anyone talks? No, I don't. Sometimes the emotional aspect of my surroundings takes the foreground, making me see everything in one particular color, like gray or jaundice yellow.

Why Factual Memory Is Safer
than Episodic Memory

Perceptions play a vital role in how a memory is stored. When it comes to narrating an episodic memory, I dare to do it only when I am very sure of my experience, as it was recorded in my mind without accessory components evolving out of my emotions or my overassociations with one component in that experience. I would never be able to forgive myself if I narrated an episodic memory, which was recorded by an overindulgence, partial indulgence, selective indulgence, or underindulgence of my senses.

Many times Mother and I have compared the same happenings and I would be surprised to find what Mother called grocery shopping was, to me, a mouthful of the taste of bitter gourd, although I was sure that bile did not fill my mouth.

I feel safer with stored answers from my factual memory because they are based on natural laws. Storing factual memory does not involve the extra component of emotion. For instance, if someone asks me the definition of *catastrophe*, I can safely say, "Catastrophe means the loss of stability in a dynamic system." I might further link the definition to the mathematics of probability in genetic mutation, which might have caused me and others like me to live with autism. To recall such a memory, I would not experience any extra colors as an additional component in the environment. My words would be directly backed by some laws in science, abiding by the rules of Nature. I would feel safer recalling such an answer than something like, "What were you doing on Thursday, when you heard the phone?"

Talking About Memories

A question may arise about how I have narrated some of my episodic memories in the early parts of my work. I have written only those selected experiences about which I knew there were witnesses. My family and friends have found me standing in front of the mirror since I was little. I did want to climb up and down the staircases in a very compulsive way. I did watch shadows and flap my hands whenever I got a chance. My learning experiences can be verified because they have the involvement of Mother, as well as my other therapists. I did not talk about those surroundings and happenings around me where I was not backed by someone who could verify it. I do not want anything to undermine the effort I put into this work.

I have analyzed my learning experiences to enable someone who is interested to realize the processes that were involved as I worked to acquire a skill. As I now work through a new skill, trying to perfect my already established abilities, I believe that there are plenty of new achievements and experiences that this body and mind will need to undergo in order to complete its life.

My body, for instance, entered its eighteenth year of life,

and the necessity to shave every day arose. How humiliating it was when Mother had to help me. I felt the need to be responsible to shave on my own. It needed to begin some day. It needed some motor planning and some motor skills to execute the plan, but that was easy because of modern technology. There are electric razors available on the market. That makes things easy.

Stories, stories one by one
With the words out they come
Stories ebb and stories swell
As I write them, them I tell.

How Do I Recall?

At some point, in some instance, my mind and body do not convey the same messages. I find my mind leading me away to some mental experience, which can be very different from what my body is supposed to experience in my physical environment. It is true that envisioning certain things allows me to remember certain facts better. But these mental experiences are far removed from the physical laws that govern those facts.

When someone in one of the laboratories where I was tested asked me how I remembered the laws of motion, I surprised her by saying that I remembered it by envisioning a brown dog chewing on the wooden handle of a hammer, sitting on a mosaic floor. That picture had nothing to do with inertia or momentum or reactions in opposite directions. A mental experience of a fact may be very different from the actual physical picture of that fact. However, certain facts may give me a closer mental picture. For example, when I became interested in trigonometric ratios, I could actually envision myself as an angle, looking at the base and the hypotenuse.

Am I in Pain?

One story flows into another while I sit with my pen in hand, looking at my written words and wondering about all the probable words I could write after these.

It is worthwhile to write about my learning how to identify and define a physical pain. To learn the sensation of physical pain, I had to mentally experience it. My mind needed to judge the location of the pain, the structure of the pain, and the nature of the pain.

Mother had to guess what caused my screams. She talked to others about it, and I heard her say, "I heard Tito falling, but he could not show me where he was hurt. I rubbed his knees, just guessing that was where he was hurt, but I saw a bump on his elbow much later."

"We need to do something about this," Mother told me. She had been discharged from the hospital after having her appendix removed, and was worried about any form of pain.

Mother began to teach me. She closed my eyes and tapped different parts of my arms and legs. She asked me to point to the body part that she had tapped. Later, I had to tell her how many times she had tapped my wrist or knee. I also had to specify whether it was the tap of a pencil or the corner of a magazine. I had to specify if it was a tap or a scratch or a rub.

Was any pain involved in those taps, scratches, or rubs? I do not know because I missed those spots initially.

Why did Mother need to close my eyes? I never missed any spot if I kept my eyes open, for I could see where she touched. I needed to know the points through touch, not vision. With more and more practice, I became much more aware of my body. I now began to be more conscious of an upset stomach or a pain in my bones. And once I felt it, I could report it to her. Mother was relieved. At least I would not die of appendicitis!

Pain includes mental pain, which can cause intense physical experiences. A torn page in a book may cause my whole body to itch. I experience terrible anxiety, which is as intense as any pain, when a schedule is disrupted. A feeling of nausea overwhelms my whole epiglottis.

What do I mean by a disrupted schedule? I have a mental map of how things should happen around me. When they do not take place as expected, the anxiety is no less than any physical pain. It produces an amplified sensation throughout my gut.

I have seen many autistic children not being able to tolerate certain types of clothes and not being able to keep their shoes on for long. Who knows what physical sensations they are experiencing at the time?

Though pain is bitter
Yet sometimes sweet
When it digs into the mind,
It shows her face
It sounds her voice
A pain of the sweetest kind.

I call one such pain a sweet pain because it brings out the best memory of a person who had once inspired my thoughts. Although now beyond my physical reach, she will forever dwell in her subtleness within my thoughts. It makes me wonder about all those lost years between us and all that lost time between us.

Where could she be?
What could she say about this?
And what could she say about that?
Would she smile at this?
Would she smile at that?
Would she be this or
Would she be that?
Since all those years
Since all that has passed?

Final Words

My autism is the dynamic experience of my relationship to the world, with its many aspects of place, people, climate, and their own interactions. I sometimes pick up on one component; other times I pick up on several components in assimilation, constantly finding how each component relates to the others, so that every situation is valued in the right way, as it is supposed to ideally be, through the challenges of my fragmented sensory experiences.

Will it be cured? There is no harm in wishing for a cure. But putting a whole amount of energy toward that wish right now may be draining and frustrating, although there are claims about finding a cure.

I have heard of doctors diagnosing a six-month-old baby as autistic and claiming to cure it within the next year! What can that claim lead to? It can make a parent wish that his child, too, had been diagnosed when he was six months old by that same doctor. And then what? What else but . . .

"Wish my Jovy was cured
Wish my worries were over

Wish Jovy led a full life
Just like any other.

But just look at Jovy
He seems not to worry
For he is playing with his shadow
Not worried about the morrow."

So what can be done with Jovy, since he is now ten, and that doctor was not around when Jovy was six months old? What else, but educate Jovy. Education is that component which brings in a meaningful relationship between the happenings around us and how our senses experience them. It helped me, and it helped many others.

Now, as I stand in front of a mirror, trying to find some inspiration for my next story, I can clearly separate the physical laws of reflection with the planes of incidence and reflection from my enchanting extrasensory experiences, leading my mind to differentiate between my alive and interactive world and the reality about what the mirror is, a mere object with a plane surface.

It is education that enabled me to record some of my experiences on paper with my pencil, so that my words might help some curious eyes that may wonder why one of his students, called Jovy, is not able to perform as well as any neuro-typical student. Or why Jovy has so much insecurity outside his familiar boundaries and abilities.

When I was very little, I remember forming wrong associations between words and objects. For instance, when I heard the word *banana* while I was looking at a cloud, I labeled the cloud "banana." Then I'd get very confused when in another instance, I looked at the cloud and someone said the word *table*. I would wonder whether some clouds were called bananas and some tables. Education helped me settle my disputes with nouns.

It was education that helped me enrich my imagination with all those probable and improbable reasonings based on science and philosophy, so that I could write my imaginings down as stories or as poetry. Education helped me to understand poetry better. It helped me understand why a few words in a phrase may be part of a poem, thus enabling me to judge my own writings, so that I can improve every work that I produce.

Many times I am asked whether I will live independently at some point in my life. My answer to that question has two approaches: an idealistic approach and a realistic approach. My idealistic approach would be that everyone needs to feel independent and self-established in this society, contributing to it, either toward its growth or its maintenance. I am part of this society, and being a member, I am no exception to this rule. So I aspire, one day, to qualify with the necessary abilities to achieve this.

Realistically, being hopeful is always good, provided I can turn those aspirations to goals to work toward. I should concentrate on my goals rather than worrying about the time spent in the process. I may achieve a goal, and I may look forward to achieving others, perhaps till the last day of my life. I may rejoice in some moments, and I may wish some moments away in the process of working toward my goals. While I work, there will be people around me, either to help me or not to help me, to judge me or not to judge me, to care about me or not to care about me, while I walk on the pathway of time through darkness and shade or light and its reflections.

Talking about independence makes me wonder, Who is truly independent in this world? A farmer who grows food is dependent on a baker, a barber, a doctor, and so on. A doctor is dependent on other people of different professions in order to survive. I am dependent and will be dependent on certain caregivers and therapists. Those caregivers and therapists need people like me to earn their bread and butter and draw their salaries. So no one is doing any favors when choosing whatever his means of livelihood is.

How independent would I be? I might ask, "How independent is he, or she, or that man on the street?" Even the universe is not independent of any of those laws that bind it together. The question of independence is a totally relative experience. We like to think that we are independent living things, forgetting how bound we are to our physical bodies, with their own packages of diseases and emotions.

What is my reason for being? What is my contribution to society? With my physical and neurological limitations, I am unable to do certain kinds of work. But I can think. And I can write. I can write down my stories on paper with my pencil. Perhaps all those stories, written and waiting to be written, will be my contribution to society. Perhaps my mere presence will be a contribution because it will remind some stray hearts that they have enough reasons to be thankful to the Maker of the Universe because they are not like me. And by my mere presence, in this form, I can remind the Creator of the Universe that all that He has created may not be perfect. And in my own striving toward the fulfillment of my existence, I can tell the Creator, I forgive Thee for every distortion in which I exist! And I am not worried about hell because I have experienced it here on earth.

Do I regret being what I am? Yes and no. Yes, from the viewpoint of my social pride, when I wonder about the humiliation I will face in the future, when I am at the mercy of others. I may overcome certain hurdles by acquiring certain skills over the years, but I may never overcome some perpetual hurdles. I may recognize, identify, and perform in certain conditions but fail to do the same in other conditions. And since every condition is so unique, learning one skill in one condition may not be applied to another. So it would be very reasonable for me to say that I do have reasons to regret. Yet there is another side of my answer, which is, "No, I do not regret." For a part of me feels comfortable with this state. When I realize my ability to interact with the shadows around me or the world of stories that appear to be forming behind a mirror, unbound by the laws of the physical world, when a little girl's giggles color the walls and ceilings with rainbow foam when she is amused by my echolalia because I am a mirror to her words, I feel blessed for being what I am.

> I am he.
> And I am me.
> I am he behind that mirror
> I am me watching the he.
> I am what.
> I am what it is to be
> Me watching the he.
> I am why.
> I am why the hell I
> Am what?

What the hell,
Is it to be?
I am the same old me.
Turning back
At the world
Watching my image in he.

As the table fan flutters my pages, I contemplate all my
written words and those which have escaped these pages.

Thus patched with stories fill this work,
Thus reflect my eyes and my ears
Through those words from my heart,
All my words from my heart.
When spins the needles of the clock
With spinning speeds of sun or earth
Through days or years, bright or dark
I spin my stories from my heart.
Thus I stray under the moon
Inside an eggshell or perhaps my room
I spin my freedom out of my doom
Inside the eggshell under the moon.
A sudden stir in some still of sleep
Wakes a moment to jump to my feet
Moments slip from the arms of the clock

Spilling time beyond my reach.
Footprints of stories they leave behind
In secret shadows, beyond time
Under the moon or the spin of the earth
I spin my words with my heart.